Get into UK
Medical School
FOR
DUMMIES®

by Dr Chris Chopdar and
Dr Neel Burton

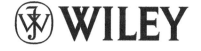

A John Wiley and Sons, Ltd, Publication

Get into UK Medical School For Dummies®

Published by:

John Wiley & Sons, Ltd
The Atrium
Southern Gate
Chichester
West Sussex
PO19 8SQ
England

www.wiley.com

© 2013 John Wiley & Sons, Ltd, Chichester, West Sussex.

Registered office

John Wiley & Sons Ltd, The Atrium, Southern Gate, Chichester, West Sussex, PO19 8SQ, United Kingdom

For details of our global editorial offices, for customer services and for information about how to apply for permission to reuse the copyright material in this book please see our website at www.wiley.com.

Wiley publishes in a variety of print and electronic formats and by print-on-demand. Some material included with standard print versions of this book may not be included in e-books or in print-on-demand. If this book refers to media such as a CD or DVD that is not included in the version you purchased, you may download this material at http://booksupport.wiley.com. For more information about Wiley products, visit www.wiley.com.

Designations used by companies to distinguish their products are often claimed as trademarks. All brand names and product names used in this book are trade names, service marks, trademarks or registered trademarks of their respective owners. The publisher is not associated with any product or vendor mentioned in this book.

For general information on our other products and services, please contact our Customer Care Department within the U.S. at 877-762-2974, outside the U.S. at (001) 317-572-3993, or fax 317-572-4002. For technical support, please visit www.wiley.com/techsupport.

A catalogue record for this book is available from the British Library.

ISBN 978-1-118-45043-7 (pbk); ISBN 978-1-118-45042-0 (ebk);
ISBN 978-1-118-45041-3 (ebk); ISBN 978-1-118-45040-6 (ebk)

10 9 8 7 6 5 4 3 2 1

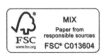

MIX
Paper from
responsible sources
FSC® C013604

WILEY

Contents at a Glance

Table of Contents

Chapter 7: Practising the UKCAT 115

Chapter 8: Breaking Down the BMAT 139

Introduction

So, you want to be a doctor. Great – clearly you love a challenge! Medicine is an exciting and varied career with interesting science underpinning clinical practice. Doctors meet a wide cross-section of society and help people through difficult times. The job can be tough, but it's also very rewarding when approached positively.

The first stage of your career is to prove to medical schools that you deserve the chance of training with them. Universities want to know that you're committed to a career in medicine and that you have a solid grasp of its rewards and challenges. They need to be certain that you can cope with the tough and unrelenting academic challenge of completing a medical degree, and they work hard to ensure that successful candidates have strong ethical awareness and good communication skills.

These varied demands mean that the application and selection process is dauntingly long and can sometimes be very frustrating. In fact, the prospect of this marathon application puts off a number of otherwise excellent candidates. So to study medicine, you need not only to have a broad range of skills, but also to be sufficiently motivated to put yourself through the application process. If you follow our advice and take things one step at a time, you can make things much easier for yourself and, hopefully, fulfill your dream of becoming a doctor.

We've been helping people get into medical school for many years. As doctors ourselves, we understand what medical schools require (and what medicine requires!), and ensure that our students know what they should be including on their applications. We also guide them through the selection tests that they face, such as the UKCAT (United Kingdom Clinical Aptitude Test) and the BMAT (Bio-Medical Admissions Test), and then help them to prepare for their interviews.

This book gives you the benefit of our accumulated experience. If you've got the talent and are prepared to put in the work, you should be well on your way to getting into medical school.

About This Book

We really want you to get into medical school; otherwise we'd have chosen a different title for this book! *Get into UK Medical School For Dummies* is aimed at intelligent, motivated people who quickly want to get to grips with a career in medicine and how to apply successfully to UK medical schools. We make this task as easy as possible, breaking down the various parts of the application process into short chapters and sections.

As well as teaching prospective medical school applicants, we're also psychiatrists and we leverage that background to show you some techniques to present yourself in the best light and cope with the stresses of the application process. These approaches help you apply successfully, and fortify you for the challenges of medical school and beyond.

In this book you find:

- ✔ Information on medicine as a career.
- ✔ What medical schools are looking for and how to acquire these skills.
- ✔ How to choose a medical school.
- ✔ How to apply to medical schools.
- ✔ How to write a compelling personal statement.
- ✔ Strategy guides and sample questions for the extra tests you may face: the UKCAT, BMAT and GAMSAT (Graduate Australian Medical School Admissions Test).
- ✔ Help on interview skills, including commonly asked questions and how to answer them.
- ✔ Some broader tips and strategies to help you navigate the sometimes confusing world of medical school applications.

Conventions Used in This Book

We don't use any strange conventions in this book. We write and arrange it as straightforwardly as possible, so that you can focus on the content. Having said that, here are a few basic conventions to be aware of:

✔ We use *italics* to highlight important words.

✔ We use **bold text** on crucial keywords in lists and to indicate correct answers in answer sections.

✔ We use this `font` for web addresses. Keep in mind that some addresses can be long, extending over two lines of text. Just ignore the line break when typing them out.

✔ We use the terms *applicant, candidate* and *student* interchangeably, and we do the same with *medical school, institution* and *university.*

What You're Not to Read

You can skip anything in sidebars – grey boxes with text in them – if you're in a rush. These boxes give you extra background information or relate a light-hearted anecdote. Taking occasional short breaks as you study is a good thing, however, and reading these sidebars helps you do just that.

Foolish Assumptions

Anyone who writes a book has to make some assumptions about the readers. In this book we assume that you want to apply to a UK university in order to study medicine. Some aspects of this process are the same in any country, and so you get some benefit even if you're applying elsewhere, but the bulk of this book is built around the assumption that you're applying to UK medical schools.

We also assume that you're prepared to put in some work. Little in life is handed to you on a plate and a place at medical school is no exception. If you want it, you need to invest time and effort.

We should mention that the sample questions we provide in this book are designed for revising applicants, to help them acquire the skills needed to answer a range of potential questions. The questions aren't designed to be used by test administrators. Also, this book focuses on an overview of the entire medical school application process so there isn't space to provide large numbers of questions for each exam. You will need to do many more practice questions than are contained here and we advise you on useful sources for these in the relevant chapters.

How This Book Is Organised

We divide this book into four parts to make the information more manageable. Most of the divisions are self-explanatory, but the information in this section helps you quickly identify the part you're looking for.

Part I: Targeting Medical School

This part introduces you to a career in medicine and how to choose and apply to medical schools. In Chapter 1 we sketch out the pros and cons of studying medicine and being a doctor. We also give you some pointers about what kind of person tends to be successful in applying to medical school. Perhaps more importantly, we think about what kind of person makes a happy, successful doctor.

In Chapter 2 we help you choose between the UK medical schools. We describe the points of difference between universities and the current funding situation in the UK. Chapter 3 provides a clear timeline for the application cycle, incorporating all the various hurdles in your way. We also point out the specific challenges that graduate and international applicants have to deal with.

Chapter 4 covers academic and non-academic entry requirements, explaining the importance of extracurricular activities and work experience. Chapter 5 is all about writing a strong personal statement for your application form. The personal statement is crucial to the shortlisting process, and so it pays dividends to focus on creating an excellent text.

Part II: Sitting the Tests

The chapters in this part describe the extra selection tests that many universities require candidates to take. In Chapter 6 we explain the UKCAT, including how and when to apply, and review its structure and timings. Chapter 7 contains a small selection of sample questions. (You can find many more practice questions in our companion book, *UKCAT For Dummies*.)

Chapters 8 and 9 review the BMAT and provide a selection of sample questions, respectively, and Chapter 10 covers the GAMSAT format.

Part III: Preparing for Interviews

This part explains the importance of interviews to the selection process and prepares you for the questions you may encounter. Chapter 11 discusses interview technique, including controlling body language and tone of voice, and Chapter 12 reviews the most common interview questions along with strategies on how to answer them effectively.

Chapter 13 contains an overview of the UK's healthcare system and some of the current challenges facing it, as well as discussing some common ethical quandaries that clinicians come across. The vast majority of newly qualified doctors commence practice in the NHS (National Health Service) and many work their entire careers in it. Medical interviewers are keen to ensure that students are going to be capable of working within its structures and so frequently ask about current controversies and the medical ethical issues that arise. This chapter prepares you for these questions.

In Chapter 14 is information on your next steps after an interview, including how to choose between offers and prepare for life at medical school. We also assess your options if you don't receive any offers.

Part IV: The Part of Tens

Every *For Dummies* book comes with a Part of Tens: sets of concise tips designed to boost your productivity. We focus on strategies to help you stand out from the crowd of applicants in Chapter 15 and provide tips to cope with the stress of applying in Chapter 16.

Icons Used in This Book

Throughout this book, we use icons in the margins that flag up important information. Here's what they mean:

This icon highlights the most important information and insights in the book. We suggest you read this material carefully.

Anyone can look up facts; our experience gives you strategic short-cuts to simplify your approach to the application process. We mark these hints in the text with this icon.

Selection processes for medical school can be tricky. This icon flags up potential pitfalls that many candidates fall into. Avoiding these mistakes dramatically improves your odds of success.

Some aspects of the selection process are underpinned by a lot of research and testing. You don't need to know this in order to get in, but understanding just why people are asking you to do things can sometimes be useful. This icon marks these explanations.

Beside this icon we include some quick exercises to make this book as practically useful for you as possible. We design them to help you get ahead of the competition, especially in areas that many candidates find tricky.

Where to Go from Here

You can read this book cover to cover for a full overview of how to get into medical school or cherry-pick those parts and chapters that address the bits you're most worried about. If you need to get on with your UCAS personal statement, turn straight to Chapter 5 now for some invaluable guidelines; if your UKCAT is fast approaching, revise the content of Chapters 6 and 7; or if you have a looming medical school interview, Part III is waiting for you to check that you're not missing anything vital.

The choice is yours; the book's structure is flexible enough to be used whichever way meets your needs the best.

For more about applying to medical school in general, further resources are on our own website (www.getintomedical school.org). And for updates about the application process (relevant dates, contact information, and so on) and changes to the tests visit us at www.dummies.com/go/getintoukmedical school.

We both wish you the very best of luck in your future career. And remember, one day we may be under your medical care, and so we have every interest in making sure that talented students succeed and get into medical school!

Part I
Targeting Medical School

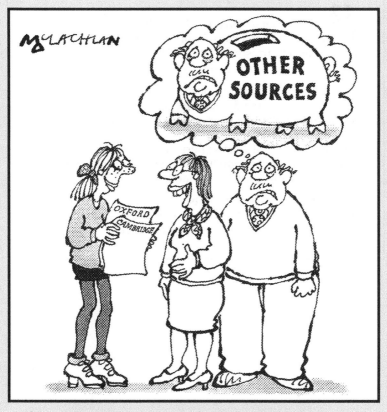

"And if you can't get enough funding from the State, there's always other sources."

In this part...

Part I is about getting to grips with the challenge of applying to medical school. The application process seems long and tiresome but breaking it down into smaller chunks makes it much easier to digest.

Your first step is making a positive choice to become a doctor. Then you need to choose some medical schools, successfully complete your application and meet the academic requirements. On top of all this, you need to get the right sort of work experience to complement your extracurricular activities in demonstrating your commitment and aptitude for medicine.

The chapters in this part cover each of these steps in turn, culminating in a chapter on how to write your application to present yourself in the best possible light.

Chapter 1

Deciding whether to Study Medicine

*M*edicine is unique. Life as a doctor is intensely rewarding and satisfying. At times, it's demanding and stressful. Applying to, and studying at medical school parallels these highs and lows. It's the start of a great adventure.

When thinking about a career as a doctor, you need to ask yourself whether you have what it takes to get into medical school and, perhaps even more importantly, whether you possess the necessary qualities to be a great doctor. In this chapter, we give you the information you need to answer these two crucial questions. We also introduce you to the system of UK medical schools and training, and onto starting your career as a doctor.

Working as a Doctor

Medicine is one of the most privileged professions to follow – as well as one of the most challenging. Applying to medical school is a serious decision. To be a good candidate, you need to understand the rewards and risks of being a doctor and make a balanced, mature decision that devoting yourself to a medical career is what you really want from life.

To help, we go through the positive and negative aspects of modern medicine, with a focus on UK practice, so you appreciate what you're getting yourself into.

Knowing the benefits

Medicine has a lot going for it as a career. It's enjoyable and the skills you learn are invaluable and highly transferable. In this section, we present some of the many upsides.

Enjoying the variety

Although some basic scheduling is involved – such as fitting professional activities around outpatient clinics and perhaps managing ward patients in hospital – one of the best aspects is the sheer variety and excitement of everyday life as a doctor. The people you see and what you do on any given day vary enormously and you meet an entire cross-section of humanity. That unpredictability is challenging but fun, and lends a certain buzz to a day's work.

You get to adapt to different situations, too, and the very act of helping other people can be highly rewarding. Dr Cox, the acerbic physician on TV's *Scrubs*, jokes that 'all doctors are praise addicts' and a kernel of truth lurks in that statement. Mind you, we'd rephrase it to say that 'doctors enjoy doing a task well, and few tasks are more worthy than being able to help when no one else can'.

Not as punchy a line, admittedly!

Relishing plenty of career options

As with many professional jobs, doctors are responsible for keeping their skills up to date and checking that their practice meets the best standards, as well as investigating and deciding upon the best way to do things. These educational, developmental, management and research or audit roles form part of a doctor's week and many medics enjoy these activities. Some doctors enjoy them so much that they form the bulk of their working lives. For example, academically-focused doctors work as university lecturers and researchers. Other doctors choose to work in the private sector, perhaps as a clinician or doing research and liaison work with pharmaceutical companies. Others still opt to work for charities, in their home country or internationally.

Some medics work on hospital management boards and in conjunction with the Department of Health or other political and lobbying organisations. A few doctors even run for elected office!

 A career in medicine offers such a wide variety of potential roles that you're almost certain to identify a niche you love. Of course, getting that ideal job can be difficult but the opportunities certainly exist.

Recognising other benefits

Although doctors don't like to talk about them much, other slightly more selfish plus points apply to being a doctor. But they're an important part of people's lives, and so we need to talk about them openly and honestly:

- ✔ **Money:** Sadly, very few doctors end up fabulously wealthy. If you want bags of money, medicine isn't the right career for you; may we suggest hedge-fund management instead? However, medicine generally offers a very comfortable income.

- ✔ **Social position:** The general public regularly place doctors highly in surveys asking people to name professions they trust and respect the most. This social status is gradually fading as the result of wider cultural changes but some of the traditional respect accorded to doctors still remains.

- ✔ **Personal identity:** Being a doctor becomes part of your identity and sense of self. From your first day at medical school you begin to discover what a doctor does, how a doctor behaves and what's expected from you. This professionalisation continues throughout your training and subsequent career and subtly alters the way you see yourself. This feeling isn't something you can easily define or shrug off, but most doctors rather like it.

Accepting the downsides

Practising medicine isn't a land of milk and honey; it has significant problems, challenges and petty hassles. When considering applying to medical school you need to come to a balanced view of whether the benefits that we describe in the preceding section outweigh the hardships.

Facing the physical and mental demands

Being a doctor can be intellectually demanding, emotionally draining and even physically exhausting. You're responsible for patients in real physical or psychological pain, and you have to deal with distraught and sometimes angry members of the public. Also, you have a lot to learn in a short space of time.

Regarding physical exhaustion, we both remember doing very long days 'on take' as junior doctors, being the first people to see sick people referred to hospital by GPs. Some days, it was so busy that we didn't get a chance to eat anything or even go to the loo. Medical life can be hectic and stressful. Even with the best will in the world, finding time to look after yourself can be tricky.

Life is now a bit easier than when we started out. European legislation reduced the number of hours junior doctors work in an average week and increased the amount of support and supervision they get from senior colleagues. However, a reduction in hours doesn't necessarily make life less stressful. If each doctor works fewer hours, they have to work more intense and antisocial shifts to ensure 24-hour clinical cover in a hospital, with fewer specialists available in a crisis situation. Moreover, without care, extra senior supervision can drift into extra bureaucracy and diminished autonomy. We write about working hours in more detail in Chapter 13, along with a discussion of all sorts of current topics and contemporary issues.

Dealing with paperwork

Bureaucracy has always been a fact of life in medicine and the NHS. But over the past 10 to 20 years, the paperwork has multiplied. The reasons are complex; the result is that administrative work takes up an ever-increasing amount of a doctor's day, often spilling over into personal time. It can be very frustrating.

 When you combine more administrative work with fewer hours of clinical work, you end up with reduced opportunities to gain experience and hone skills. This situation can lead to doctors with insufficient experience working outside the scope of their competence. The consequences are potentially lethal for patients and some systems have been put into place to prevent this problem, but systems are rarely perfect.

Developing patience

Medicine, especially in the NHS, can be quite hierarchical. Advancing to the next grade ahead of a pre-determined schedule is difficult, regardless of your talent. The NHS features a definite element of having to serve time. This time can be instrumental to gaining experience, but remaining patient can be tough. Applicants to medical school are naturally highly aspirational, keen to step up to the next level. To progress in medicine you need to temper that positive drive with copious amounts of patience.

You also need patience and persistence to cope with endless exams and appraisal. As we relate in Chapters 6 to 10, you may need to take tests even to be shortlisted for a university interview, and the application process is almost one year long. Medical school itself generally lasts five or six years and is crammed full of more tests, culminating in medical finals. Later, you sit Royal College exams for your chosen area of specialisation, spanning yet more years. And after that come annual appraisals of professional development and five-yearly revalidations of your fitness to practise medicine. Sometimes, the regulatory burden seems immense and unfair.

We don't discuss these downsides to put you off medicine, and you do receive training to mitigate the impact of many of these difficulties. We just want you to be aware of them so that they don't hit you like a freight train when you start.

Being aware of the downsides allows you to make a balanced decision about being a doctor. It also helps you explain that choice during the medical school selection process, such as when writing your personal statement and answering questions during interviews (check out Chapters 5 and 12, respectively).

Succeeding as a Doctor

Doctors share some key individual traits. These personal qualities are refined during training but can't be wholly taught. As a result, medical schools try to select candidates who show signs of possessing them.

No one can consistently display all these necessary qualities and naturally some people are stronger in some areas and weaker in others. Medical schools don't expect perfection; they want potential.

We now detail some of these desired characteristics, such as enjoying dealing with people and continuing to learn, making stress work for you and having a strong ethical foundation. When you know what makes a good doctor, you can decide whether you measure up, and also tailor your upcoming work experience and extracurricular activities to highlight these qualities. Turn to Chapter 4 to find out more about what medical schools look for in applicants.

Liking people and communicating well

Liking people is a crucial prerequisite to being a good doctor. Medicine isn't just science; it blends scientific knowledge with wisdom and humanity in order to improve quality of life. You meet people every day and if you don't like them, you're going to find fulfilling this requirement difficult.

Liking people manifests differently depending on personality. Very basically, an extrovert doctor may feel energised by talking to others and working in a team, whereas an introvert may get a similar buzz from observing situations, figuring out what makes people tick and how to influence situations positively. For an interesting take on these different qualities, check out the sidebar 'Inward looking or outgoing?'

Both introverts and extroverts can be great doctors. One type isn't better than the other and medical schools like to train a range of different people to become doctors. You need to understand how you relate to other people and use that self-knowledge to improve your communication skills. It's about using your natural tendencies to your best advantage and, of course, to that of your patients.

You don't have to be loud and sociable in order to prove that you like people. In fact, some of the loudest people probably don't like others; they may well just like the sound of their own voice!

As well as liking people, doctors need to communicate effectively with them. Some studies suggest that patients forget about 80 per cent of what a doctor says, but this isn't necessarily the doctor's fault. A medical consultation can be nerve-wracking and that distraction can impair a patient's memory.

Good communication skills limit the damage by ensuring that patients feel heard and understand what you're talking about.

Some people are natural communicators. They know when to talk and when to be silent. Their innate empathy and intuition gives them the knack of judging what other people may be thinking. Placing yourself in someone else's shoes and guessing what they're thinking is called *theory of mind*. People with good theory of mind are potentially great communicators. Most people aren't this naturally talented, but practice helps improve communication skills.

The key is to consciously consider what other people may be worried about. Suppose you want to stay out late at a party but your parents insist on a curfew of midnight. Put yourself in their shoes; what are they concerned about? It's unlikely to be the time itself. The time is a proxy marker for a range of other worries about what you might get up to if given too much leeway.

Arguing about the time is therefore unlikely to result in a later curfew. If anything, it will make your parents more concerned about what you might be planning. Instead, a more appropriate strategy would be to reassure them about your plans. Give them information about where you'll be, who you'll be with and what you'll be doing. Tell them you'll give them a call at some point during the evening to check in (and stick to that promise). You might not get an extended curfew this time, but by addressing the actual concerns rather than an arbitrary time limit, you're far more likely to build up enough trust to get it lifted next time.

Inward looking or outgoing?

Psychiatrist Carl Jung, drawing on playwright-philosopher Friedrich Schiller's fertile correspondence with the poet Goethe, suggested that the conscious mind of the introvert is driven largely by the ego (the internal sense of self) while their sense of relatedness (emotional response) to objects in the external world is diminished.

By contrast, the extrovert is captivated by the world and their relationship to it, with the ego secondary to this. Jung said that 'the extrovert discovers himself in the fluctuating and the changeable; the introvert in the constant.' Emotional experience is 'positively painful' to the extreme introvert but for the extrovert 'it must on no account be missed'.

No statement better illustrates this difference than when introverted Schiller wrote to the extrovert Goethe: 'You have a kingdom to rule and I only a somewhat numerous family of ideas which I would like to expand into a little universe.'

Formal personality tests exist to determine whether you're an introvert or extrovert and it can be fun and revealing to take them. But most reasonably insightful people will be able to read Schiller's statement and correctly intuit which group they belong to. Once you know that, you can begin to work on developing your communication skills and optimise your chances of getting into medical school and being a good doctor.

That's a small practical example of how theory of mind gets you positive results. And notice that not only did you get something out of it, but so did your parents. Negotiations succeed because both sides win something, not because one side wins the argument and the other loses.

You can develop theory of mind in lots of little ways.

Next time you're sitting in a café, take time to subtly study other patrons. Try to guess what they're doing there, what the relationship is with the other people they're talking to, what sort of place they work at and what they might be feeling or thinking. You may even be able to hear enough of their conversation to check whether your guesses were right.

Of course, don't be intrusive or rude. We're talking about being an active observer of life, not becoming a nosy-parker!

Medical schools are very keen to select candidates with excellent communication skills (and look for and may directly question you about it in the interview, as we describe in Chapters 11 and 12).

Coupled with academic ability, effective communication is a potent predictor of being suited to medicine. It greatly reduces the odds of doctors receiving complaints; most such proceedings stem from misunderstanding, confusion and hurt feelings rather than mal-practice.

The other great advantage of good communication skills is that they let you adapt to dealing with different kinds of people. Doctors meet a wide cross-section of the public, both as patients and as colleagues. Being good with people helps you fit in smoothly, making your job much easier.

To find out more about good communication skills and how you can develop these, pick up a copy of *Communication Skills For Dummies* by Elizabeth Kuhnke (Wiley).

Enjoying intellectual activity

You don't need to be a genius to be a doctor, but you do need to be able to absorb vast quantities of information accurately and rapidly. For that task, having an excellent memory allied to good organisational skills and an inquisitive, logical mind is extremely helpful.

A strong science inclination is important, especially for dealing with the first couple of years of medical school. After that, you'll have a lot of scientific knowledge to memorise but you start to problem solve as well, which is when being logical comes in very handy. A lot of clinical practice depends on spotting similarities and differences to situations you've already been in.

Take the case of someone coming into the Accident and Emergency Department (A&E) with chest pain. Modern medicine instantly invokes a barrage of investigations to diagnose the cause, but a good doctor is simultaneously narrowing down the potential different causes of the chest pain through questioning and examining patients and mentally comparing the data to previous cases. For more on this type of problem-solving, take a look at the nearby sidebar 'Introducing algorithms and heuristics'.

Problem-solving skills can be improved. Any activity that encourages lateral thinking and decision making is likely to improve your ability to solve problems. An example is the positive effect that familiarity and practice has on exam performance. But unrelated activities can also boost cerebral skills like pattern recognition, deduction and lateral thinking. Activities as diverse as crossword or riddle solving, chess, art and debating all encourage the development of these skills.

Introducing algorithms and heuristics

The approach to problem-solving that we discuss in this section is called the *hypo-thetico-deductive model.* Results of investigations are slotted into this framework, confirming or denying the initial hypothesis, ultimately enabling a heuristically-derived solution, and means doctors can spot rare cases where an algorithm alone may be insufficient.

Algorithms are well-defined, consistent protocols for carrying out a task; essentially, they're a series of specific instructions. For example, if you use satellite navigation to get to a destination, you follow the sequence of spoken instructions precisely to complete your journey. Many employers require their employees to follow strictly algorithmic processes. A factory assembly line is the archetypal example but many office workers also work the same way.

Heuristics are the techniques used to derive a solution; because they're not set in stone, they can be wrong. Imagination and lateral thinking are harnessed to interpret incoming data and weigh up its meaning. A doctor has to think in this way to be most effective.

Evidence-based medicine has resulted in an increasing number of manuals and protocols that follow pure algorithmic approaches. Paradoxically, this explosion in the number of available algorithms means that heuristic thinking is more important than ever. A doctor has to juggle all these different protocols and decide which are most pertinent to their patient. But they also need to justify decisions clearly and logically in the medical record, and so the best doctors possess an unusual combination of analytical and lateral thinking.

Thriving on stress

Make no mistake, practising medicine can be stressful: the antisocial hours, the administrative burden of the job and the challenge of working with the very ill.

Doctors understand that stress is a natural response to difficult situations and can be channelled positively. Stress can encourage hard work, courage and dedication. Without any stress at all staying motivated can be difficult. If stress levels rise too high, however, mistakes happen. Concentration slips and people become distracted and exhausted. Therefore, taking time out from medicine to relax and recharge is important.

Think back to the last time you felt stressed and try to remember the emotions and sensations you felt. Most people recognise acute stress as a combination of rapid shallow breathing, racing pulse, pounding heart and sometimes even sweatiness, nausea and tremor. More long-term stress makes you feel tense, anxious and as if the weight of the world is on your shoulders.

> ## Becoming optimally aroused
>
> We're afraid this sidebar is a little less interesting than the above heading may suggest! It's about discovering how to balance stress so that it works for you.
>
> The Yerkes–Dodson law describes the relationship between arousal and performance. Named after the two psychologists who codified it, it states that performance increases as physiological and mental excitement increases, but only up to a point. Beyond this, the state of arousal becomes increasingly detrimental to performance. The relationship between arousal and performance is therefore an inverted-U.
>
> The optimal level of arousal varies depending on the task at hand but the real skill is in knowing yourself well enough to gauge whether you're operating at peak efficiency or whether stress is causing bad decisions and poor performance. It's a skill that improves over time. For now, try to think back to situations where you were worried about a task and then used that energy to achieve beyond your expectations. That's what optimal arousal feels like.
>
> Accepting the Yerkes–Dodson law can stop you from overworking and keep you practising medicine safely. Cases of medical negligence can result from slipshod errors brought about by stress and exhaustion.

Stress arises because of a mismatch between our future and our current situations. Acute stress results in flowing adrenaline, which boosts our energy levels and ability to concentrate. Chronic stress is less helpful, fuelling distress and unhappiness.

Managing chronic stress levels through relaxation and distraction exercises while using acute stress to keep you energised and productive is crucial. To understand stress more deeply, check out the sidebar 'Becoming optimally aroused'. For more about coping with stress, check out Chapter 16.

Being reliable and trustworthy

People's lives depend on doctors. They have to be reliable, which means being organised, punctual and conscientious. Keeping your promises and not making ones that you can't keep are equally essential.

Doctors have to maintain the highest standards of personal integrity. When you work with the most vulnerable members of society, the opportunities for abusing that trust are plentiful. We don't think anyone goes into medicine to abuse people but life proves that originally good people sometimes end up doing bad things. The process is usually gradual, with one thing leading to another.

Are you a good person?

In Plato's *Republic*, one of Socrates's interlocutors suggests that morality is merely a social construction stemming from the desire to maintain a good reputation and avoid punishment. If those sanctions are removed, the questioner suggests, moral character would evaporate. He uses the example of the mythological Ring of Gyges to support his argument. According to legend, the shepherd Gyges uses a magical invisibility ring to seduce a queen. With her help, he murders her husband and takes the throne.

Plato, speaking through Socrates in the text, disagrees, replying that a higher form of justice exists. He suggests that the man who doesn't abuse power feels in control of himself, and is therefore happier.

Regardless of whether it's in response to higher inner purpose, or mere fear of the General Medical Council, we advise that you take a just approach to clinical practice!

Being mindful of the potential long-term negative impact of your actions operates as a powerful restraint against the temptation of such 'slippery slope' actions.

Studying Medicine: Medical School and Beyond

Attending medical school can be a daunting and confusing prospect, but it's also enjoyable and exciting. In this section we provide an overview of medical school. You can find more details on selecting schools in Chapter 2, planning your application in Chapter 3 and doing the groundwork to apply in Chapter 4.

Currently, 32 medical schools operate in the UK and we list them in Table 1-1 along with details of the different degrees they award. Some are standalone institutions while others form part of universities that also teach other subjects. The table contains 34 entries rather than 32, because Durham and Lancaster don't confer their own degrees: other universities do that for them. All these medical schools are recognised by the GMC (the General Medical Council), the regulator that licenses doctors to practise medicine.

From August 2013, Peninsula College of Medicine and Dentistry splits into two new medical schools: University of Exeter Medical School, and Plymouth University Peninsula Schools of Medicine and Dentistry. From October 2013, applicants will be able to select either or both of these schools.

Students who successfully complete medical school are awarded medical degrees, with the exact degree title varying between universities. The most common is the MBBS (Bachelor of Medicine, Bachelor of Surgery) but variations exist such as the University of Oxford's BM BCh, where the 'Ch' stands for Chirurgery (an archaic word for surgery).

Table 1-1	UK Medical Schools
Medical School	*Medical Degree Awarded*
University of Aberdeen School of Medicine	MBChB (Bachelor of Medicine, Bachelor of Surgery)
Barts and The London School of Medicine and Dentistry	MBBS (Bachelor of Medicine, Bachelor of Surgery)
University of Birmingham Medical School	MBChB
Brighton and Sussex Medical School	BMBS (Bachelor of Medicine, Bachelor of Surgery)
Bristol Medical School	MBChB
School of Clinical Medicine, University of Cambridge	MB BChir (Bachelor of Medicine, Bachelor of Surgery)
Cardiff University School of Medicine	MBBCh (Bachelor of Medicine, Bachelor of Surgery)
Durham University School of Medicine and Health	Pre-clinical only; degrees awarded by Newcastle University
Dundee Medical School	MBChB
University of Edinburgh Medical School	MBChB
Glasgow Medical School	MBChB
Hull York Medical School	MBBS
Imperial College School of Medicine	MBBS
Keele University School of Medicine	MBChB
King's College London School of Medicine and Dentistry	MBBS

Medical School	Medical Degree Awarded
Lancaster Medical School	Degrees awarded by Liverpool University
Leeds School of Medicine	MBChB
Leicester Medical School	MBChB
Liverpool Medical School	MBChB
London School of Hygiene and Tropical Medicine	MSc (Master of Science: postgraduate/intercalating students only)
Manchester Medical School	MBChB
Newcastle University Medical School	MBBS
Norwich Medical School/ University of East Anglia	MBBS
University of Nottingham Medical School	BMBS
Medical Sciences Division, University of Oxford	BM BCh (Bachelor of Medicine, Bachelor of Surgery)
Peninsula College of Medicine and Dentistry	BMBS
Queen's University Belfast Medical School	MB BCh BAO (BAO stands for *Baccalaureus in Arte Obstetricia*, that is, Bachelor of Obstetrics)
Sheffield Medical School	MBChB
Southampton Medical School	BM
University of St Andrews School of Medicine	Pre-clinical BSc only; clinical training degrees conferred by partner universities
St George's, University of London	MBBS
Swansea University School of Medicine	MBBCh (graduate entry only)
UCL Medical School	MBBS
Warwick Medical School	MBChB

The GMC considers these degrees to be equivalent and they all permit you to register provisionally as a doctor. After successfully gaining enough experience in very junior posts (Foundation Year 1), doctors are eligible for full GMC registration. They then work across a range of specialities during their Foundation Year 2, before opting to specialise in a specific field or general practice.

Specialisation involves Core Training, during which you complete the relevant Royal College exams and Higher Training. At the end of this multi-year process you get the qualifications you need to apply for consultant jobs in the National Health Service (NHS). GP training works in a similar way. You can find more information about specialising in the 'Training after you're a doctor' section of Chapter 13.

The majority of students enter medical school as undergraduates, after completing secondary education. Medical school typically lasts five years but some universities allow you to intercalate a second degree (typically a BSc: Bachelor of Science) at the cost of another year's study. Intercalating students thereby leave medical school with two degrees. We describe intercalated degrees in Chapter 2.

Traditionally, medical schools divided their training between pre-clinical and clinical courses. Oxford, Cambridge and St Andrews still maintain this separation of pre-clinical and clinical work:

- ✔ **Pre-clinical training** involves a thorough grounding in the basic sciences such as anatomy and physiology (see the nearby sidebar 'Studying the basic sciences' for a fuller list).

- ✔ **Clinical training** involves working directly with patients in hospitals or other similar locations.

The remaining medical schools offer *integrated* courses, in which pre-clinical and clinical training isn't strictly divided. You start working in hospitals from your first year of medical school. Both training systems have their advantages; we cover this topic in much more detail in Chapter 2.

In addition, differences apply in the way medical schools deliver the course content. They all use a variety of teaching methods, from lectures to small group work, but the emphasis and relative proportions vary between schools. Also, an increasing number of medical schools offer accelerated training programmes for graduate applicants. These are usually only four years long, but cover the same curriculum as the undergraduate courses.

Studying the basic sciences

Basic sciences form the scientific backbone of medical practice. Examples include:

✓ Anatomy: The study of the physical structure of the body

✓ Biochemistry: The chemistry taking place in the body

✓ Cytology and Histology: The studies of individual cells and tissues

✓ Genetics: The study of genes

✓ Immunology: How the immune system functions

✓ Microbiology: The study of bacteria, viruses and other pathogens

✓ Neuroscience: The study of the nervous system, including the brain

✓ Pharmacology: How drugs work

✓ Physiology: How the body functions

Graduate entry medicine is very demanding, both in terms of the pace of the course and the difficulty of winning a place. You can find more information about graduate entry medicine in Chapter 3.

Medical school also offers a huge number of opportunities outside of your medical training, including clubs, societies and sports teams catering for almost every passion and ability. This is especially true at those medical schools that are part of larger universities.

Undoubtedly medical school involves a lot of hard work, but most doctors look back on their time at university with a great deal of affection. You do a lot of growing up, develop a myriad of new skills and get to go to places and do things you'd never do otherwise.

The whole experience is really a lot of fun, even if it does make you feel like pulling your hair out at times. And that combination makes it about as good a preparation for being a doctor as you can get!

Chapter 2

Choosing a Medical School

In This Chapter

▶ Deciding what kind of medical school suits you

▶ Applying to Oxbridge

▶ Paying your way

Selecting a medical school that's right for you can be a difficult decision. The websites and prospectuses all proudly proclaim wonderful teaching, vibrant social opportunities, beautiful settings and vast quantities of money raining down from the heavens in the form of student funding.

Separating fact from fiction (sorry, we mean 'generous interpretation of reality') can be tricky. The truth is that all UK medical schools are excellent institutions of higher learning and they all provide a good well-rounded medical education. After you graduate, beyond your first couple of jobs, which medical school you attended rarely matters.

But medical schools aren't interchangeable. On the contrary, large differences can exist. Choosing between them involves deciding what's important to you rather than ranking them according to a grand unified scale. You can get an idea of what medical schools offer by talking to past and present students and visiting universities on their open days. Doing so gives you a feel for what studying and socialising at a particular medical school is like. Each medical school runs at least one open day per year and typically more, so make the effort to visit the ones you're interested in.

To help you make a decision, we cover some of the key differentiating factors between medical schools – including the vital subject of teaching style and methods – and take a closer look at Oxbridge universities, and the thorny issue of funding.

Weighing Up the Various Factors

To choose between medical schools, you need to think practically, considering aspects such as where you want to live, what teaching methods you prefer and more. We believe that these are the crucial aspects to consider rather than focusing too closely on statistics.

Understanding the limitations of statistics

Most prospective medical students spend hours poring over tables, comparing applicant-to-place ratios, looking up statistics online and generally seeking a perfect application strategy. In addition, many websites and books about medical schools devote inordinate amounts of space to the minutiae of application statistics, breaking them down by course, institution, region and more. To put it simply: we don't.

We think that application statistics are so misleading as to be actively unhelpful to you. If you spend more than five minutes looking at application statistics before applying to study medicine, you're wasting your time.

In our opinion only one statistic has even borderline utility: in 2011, 21,726 people applied to study at medical schools. Of these applicants, 7,798 people were accepted, making the overall applicant-to-acceptance ratio approximately 2.8:1. In other words, only about 36 per cent of applicants received at least one offer.

This statistic gives you a rough idea of the intense competition for places across both undergraduate and graduate entry courses. Graduate entry is even more competitive and undergraduate entry slightly less so.

But even this simple percentage has a serious problem as a thought experiment illustrates. Consider your own position: you're deciding whether to apply to medical school. You look at the overall application ratio of 2.8 and decide that this means you have approximately a 36 per cent chance of getting in. But that's not the case.

The 36 per cent figure is based on those who actually apply, not those who simply *consider* applying. This difference matters because more people consider applying than actually apply. If you're reading this book before you submit your application, you aren't formally part of the population from which the statistic is derived. Therefore it doesn't apply to you!

Lies, damn lies and statistics

Statistics are even more unhelpful at institution level. For example, applicant ratios at individual institutions are much higher than 2.8. They range from about 7 to around 14, which gives the impression that medical school is much harder to get into than is the case. The distortion occurs because a single applicant to medicine can apply to up to four institutions in an application cycle. But each of these applicants can only occupy one eventual place at medical school. So the high applicant ratio for individual medical schools is unrealistic.

This situation is further exacerbated by some institutions appearing easier or harder to get into than they really are. For instance, Brighton and Sussex Medical School routinely has significantly more applicants per place than Oxford does. So is getting into Brighton and Sussex harder? No. Brighton and Sussex has an artificially high application ratio because it's a vibrant town in a pleasant part of the country. Oxford has an artificially low ratio because many applicants see it as a place where only the best can get in and so dare not apply. While the average applicant to Brighton and Sussex is fairly similar to the overall population of medical school applicants, the average applicant to Oxford is of a higher calibre.

In addition, there's also the problem of differential rates of acceptance. Almost everyone who gets an offer from Oxford accepts it, but the proportion of offer acceptances is lower for Brighton. This is compounded by people receiving offers from both Oxford and Brighton: they select Oxford as their firm acceptance and Brighton as their insurance offer, and later go on to meet Oxford's offer.

UCAS and institutions gather this kind of data partly because it's very easy to collect, but mostly because it can be used to guide the future of medical education. Experts can analyse it to spot trends, anticipate future supply and demand, determine whether universities are hitting social inclusiveness targets and so on. In other words, the data are useful for generating statistics to monitor population-level trends, but far less useful to you as an individual candidate.

Statistics are able to give you information only about the overall population. If the population is *homogenous* – all members of the population are sufficiently similar – you can use the statistics to tell you something about individual members of the group too. But applicants to medical school are definitely not homogenous. Some have higher grades, or better UKCAT/BMAT scores, or more work experience, or more suitable personalities than others. Therefore they don't all share the same chance of getting into medical school. Some have a far greater chance of getting an offer than 36 per cent and others a far lower one.

Bias, chance and confounding

Interpreting statistical information is a key part of modern medical education. The average layperson has a dreadful understanding of statistics, probabilities and risk, whereas medicine requires a firm grasp of these concepts to understand scientific studies and apply or explain them correctly to patients.

The first step is deciding whether a set of statistics is relevant to your needs. In other words, do you match the population the statistics refer to, and are the statistics about a topic you're interested in? If the answer to either question is no, the statistics have no direct relevance to you and any conclusions you draw from them may be inaccurate.

If the statistics are potentially relevant, you then have to decide if they have *validity*: are the figures sound enough to be trustworthy?

Three things undermine causal conclusions drawn from statistics: chance (where the link you're considering is down to sheer luck), bias (a systematic difference exists in the population being studied and the one you're interested in) and confounding variables (another factor independently influences the outcome).

In this section, you can see that we demonstrate that application statistics have potential shortcomings across all three areas, which is why we suggest giving them only fleeting attention.

In essence, applying to medical schools is a competitive process and not a lottery where your personal odds reflect those of the general population. Looking at application ratios is pointless because they tell you almost nothing about your *personal* chances of getting into medical school.

Instead of spending hours pondering application data, spend your time checking the entry requirements, studying for your exams, practising for the application exams, getting work experience, improving your interview skills and so on. In fact, do anything that really improves your individual odds of getting into medical school!

Living where you want

Location, location, location may be the estate agent's mantra, but it also applies to choosing a medical school. Think about this: you're probably going to be at the same medical school for five or six years. That's a pretty big chunk out of your life; do you want to spend it in a place you hate?

You can group UK medical schools into three sets of locations: London, other urban centres, and provincial or relatively rural. Some pretty big differences in your potential lifestyle exist between those three destinations. In addition, don't forget that you can study overseas as well.

Choosing London

London is a world city. It's immense, even compared to other major British cities, and has an unparalleled diversity of accommodation, leisure options and patient groups. These factors can make it very attractive as a study location, especially for those who've never lived in the capital.

London also has significant downsides, however. It's a large and frequently anonymous city that can feel alienating and overwhelming. Transport links can be frustrating, especially when you're rushing from one part of the city to another to attend an outpatient clinic or lecture. Parts of London can be quite grimy; anyone who's travelled on the Tube and later blown his nose only to see black phlegm emerge can attest to this! And if your budget is tight, expect to feel the strain of the high living costs of the capital.

How you view the benefits against the downsides depends on your personality and what you want from your time at university. London is unquestionably an exciting city but its 24/7 buzz can lead to feelings of hopelessness and loss of purpose.

Selecting other urban locations

The medical schools set in Britain's other major urban centres – such as Manchester and Liverpool – generally offer a less sprawling version of London. They're also less cosmopolitan than the capital, but transport is more straightforward and accommodation costs more reasonable. They benefit from good links with regional hospitals and often have opportunities to study there for part of your training, which adds breadth to your experience.

Getting out of town

Medical schools based in provincial towns and more rural settings are very different beasts. Institutions such as Nottingham and Peninsula tend to be in quieter locations, with a narrower patient base. Leisure opportunities are more focused on the student population, which can lead to a more tightly knit student body. Your placements are likely to include stints at a number of different clinical bases across the county, and so having a car and being able to drive is a great help.

Oxford and Cambridge (and to some extent, St Andrews) can be considered as special cases of the provincial medical schools. They have uniquely ancient histories and correspondingly high international prestige as centres of learning. Applying to Oxford and Cambridge creates additional hurdles; check out the 'Aiming at Oxbridge' section later in this chapter for more details.

Studying abroad

UK candidates can study medicine outside the UK. This option is good if you plan to work in another country after qualifying, or you don't mind the costs associated with private medical schools and then return to practise in the UK after completing any necessary qualification conversion formalities.

Historically, high fees deterred UK medical applicants from applying abroad, but the changing tuition fee structure in the UK is making foreign universities look more attractive. Fees are still higher than in the UK but the difference is less.

If you're fluent in another language, you can potentially study in any university in that country, but even if you're fluent only in English, you still have some options abroad.

The European Union (EU) can be an attractive choice because no further conversion exam is required if you return to the UK to practise after qualifying. Examples of EU medical schools that teach in English include Maastricht University in the Netherlands (you need to speak Dutch if you want to carry on there for your clinical training) and Charles University in Prague (although the entrance procedure is conducted in Czech).

Outside of the EU, you may like the idea of studying medicine somewhere sunny. For example, St Matthew's University School of Medicine is in the British Cayman Islands.

If you apply to a foreign university, be sure that you can pay the fees because you won't receive funding through the UK system. For example, St Matthew's charges about US$100,000 for its four-year medical course and that's at the cheaper end of the spectrum. We discuss fees in more detail in the section titled 'Funding Your Place'.

You need to research foreign medical schools carefully to understand how their application process works and whether their qualification is internationally recognised. The General Medical Council (GMC) keeps a list of foreign medical schools whose qualifications it accepts, as well as those from which it requires extra evidence. Check out the relevant page on the GMC's website (www.gmc-uk. org/doctors/registration_applications/acceptable_ primary_medical_qualification.asp).

Learning in the way you prefer

Medical schools pride themselves on offering students a top-flight educational experience. They spend a lot of time refining their courses, researching teaching methods and selecting faculty who can deliver their vision of medical education. As a result, each medical school is unique. Some are at the extremes of a teaching style and others lean heavily towards one model in some respects but in a different direction in others.

 Significant ideological differences exist among medical schools and so choose carefully and accordingly; specific medical courses reward students who are aware of their personal preferred learning style.

In this section, we guide you through what's on offer by breaking down the key differences in teaching styles and methods, so that you can decide which environment suits you best.

 Think of medical education as possessing several different dimensions and each medical school occupying a slightly different position within this theoretical multi-dimensional space.

Teaching styles

In essence, UK medical schools use two different teaching styles: traditional subject-based courses and integrated courses. The latter can be subject-based or systems-based.

Twenty-five years ago, all medical school courses were traditional and subject-based – and a few still are:

- ✔ **Traditional courses** clearly delineate pre-clinical and clinical training:
    - *Pre-clinical* training focuses heavily on the basic sciences, with minimal patient contact.
    - *Clinical* training teaches you to apply that knowledge to health-related problems.
- ✔ **Subject-based courses** study each science (such as anatomy or physiology) separately.

This clear separation between pre-clinical and clinical years has advantages. Students can focus on the science without being distracted by having to adapt to working in a hospital or clinic. In many respects the course resembles doing an intensive undergraduate multi-disciplinary science degree.

This division appeals to academically-inclined students with strong science backgrounds and highly structured minds; in other words, people who like to complete one task successfully before moving on to another.

The downside of traditional subject-based courses is that your clinical years come as a bit of a culture shock. You're plunged straight into the hurly-burly of hospital wards, seeing patients, and can feel remarkably de-skilled, as if all that pre-clinical science knowledge is suddenly irrelevant. Of course, as you get up to speed with how medicine works in practice, all that science knowledge begins to fall into place and create a strong foundation for sound clinical practice. But the change between pre-clinical and clinical years is striking.

In an attempt to minimise this marked difference, some schools started introducing integrated courses around 20 years ago. In *integrated courses,* medical students have some exposure to actual patients from the start of their pre-clinical years.

Some schools have only limited integration; perhaps a day of clinical involvement a month. But others are so integrated that it's not always clear when pre-clinical years end and clinical years begin.

Integrated courses do some things very well. They encourage students to begin applying their core scientific education to clinical practice from an early stage. This clinical involvement can identify communication or other soft-skill deficits early on, giving students and teachers plenty of time to remedy them. And they can motivate students by making medicine seem more real.

The flipside is that a first year pre-clinical medical student can feel a bit of a gooseberry on a hospital ward. Although a student just starting his clinical years in a traditional course can also feel lost, at least he's had the benefit of a strong scientific education. Perhaps more importantly, the extra years of study before seeing patients add to his experience and maturity, and lend a balanced perspective on life. The first year, a pre-clinical student on an integrated course, however, has none of this extra life experience. Medical schools recognise this potential problem with integrated courses and try to ensure close supervision and training to help students through this period.

Some integrated courses are subject-based, as traditional courses always are, but they can also be systems-based.

Systems-based courses approach learning about the body differently. Instead of focusing on different scientific disciplines (anatomy, biochemistry, physiology and so on), they focus on the different elements of the body (the heart, the lungs, the gut and so on). You learn the relevant basic sciences through this systems-based focus.

The idea is to get students thinking about the body as a practical set of interacting systems that can go wrong, that impact on each other and that drugs or surgery can modify.

Making definitive statements about whether traditional or integrated courses are better is difficult, because they come down to your personal preference and strengths. Our view is that:

- Traditional subject-based courses offer a stronger foundation in the basic sciences. They suit you if you have strong science leanings, prefer focusing on one thing at a time and don't mind waiting a couple of years before seeing patients.

- Integrated courses, especially systems-based ones, suit you if you're keen to start seeing patients soon and prefer taking a medical and patient-orientated approach right from the start of your training.

Teaching methods

Within the two teaching styles that we describe in the preceding section – traditional and integrated courses – different teaching methods are used.

In the traditional method of medical education, lectures and practical experiments are the most common teaching methods during pre-clinical training (closely paralleling typical undergraduate pure science courses). The clinical years are essentially an apprenticeship in which students observe what doctors do, try it under their supervision, and then help others learn in the same way (the 'see one, do one, teach one' method).

Not all students thrive within this framework. Some find lectures boring and are unable to focus consistently during them. This situation isn't necessarily a problem in itself, provided those students work independently to learn the content. However, it makes the overall learning experience inefficient.

As a result, all medical schools now employ more modern teaching methods. The more traditional schools use them to augment a lecture programme, while others have replaced lectures entirely. These new methods tend to be more interactive and iterative than lectures. Students actively think around a topic to answer questions and explore or test concepts.

Changing cultures

If you'll forgive us a little politically-incorrect honesty, in the old days it didn't matter that lectures are a fairly inefficient teaching method because students who found particular lectures (or lecturers) unrewarding simply skipped them. They learnt what they needed in their own time, restoring efficiency to their medical education . . . and enjoying the occasional lie-in! The flipside was that if you were cheeky and did this frequently, you implicitly took on full personal responsibility for your potential failure.

These days medical schools aggressively monitor their students' movements with innovations such as having to sign class attendance sheets. If students have less scope to choose their own preferred learning environment, medical schools implicitly accept a greater responsibility to be effective and efficient in their teaching methods.

The reasons for this cultural change are complex and reflect different outlooks by both medical schools and students. Medical schools increasingly need to justify their funding to their parent universities and indirectly to central government. They need to be seen to be proactive in teaching and in identifying struggling students. And their reputation partly depends on ensuring very high pass rates.

Students too are more demanding nowadays. They pay whopping tuition fees and naturally expect a high-quality education in return. An inefficient educational experience is no longer acceptable to them as consumers.

The changed relationship between medical schools and their students reflects a much broader cultural shift in society between providers and consumers of services, towards litigiousness and apportioning of blame.

Doctors need to be aware of these societal changes because they also affect how patients view them. The same trends result in increased risk aversion and defensive medicine, all at the potential cost of unnecessary and even harmful interventions.

The most 'extreme' medical schools subscribe wholly to the problem-based learning (PBL) method. Here, teachers pose students a broad question, for example 'What is a heart attack?'. Students then work with each other and the teacher to develop answers. This work can include devising new relevant questions such as 'What kinds of heart attack are there?' or 'What happens to heart muscle when it no longer gets enough oxygenated blood?'.

The idea behind the PBL method is that students are required to work with each other in an inquisitive way to encourage the development of problem-solving skills alongside learning new facts. Research suggests that this method is quite effective in the long-term, even if it may at first seem partial and unsystematic.

Other more intermediate forms of non-lecture learning include class-based discussions where the teacher takes the lead in setting the course of the learning activity; tutorials where very small groups of students discuss a topic together with their tutor; and seminars, which are somewhere in-between these two methods.

Medical schools also use practical classes to teach some skills, and some still use cadaver dissection to teach anatomy. With fewer people leaving their bodies to medical science, and the increasing cost of running these classes and the better availability of computer-animated 3D modelling, such dissection is on the decline. As a replacement, some schools use *prosection,* in which an experienced anatomist dissects the relevant body-part and demonstrates the 3D anatomy to medical students.

Choosing your preferred teaching approach

Most medical schools use a variety of teaching styles and methods and don't adopt a single extreme style. Therefore, being precise about different schools' styles and methods is difficult – and unhelpful. We can state the following, however:

- ✔ Oxford, Cambridge and St Andrews generally adopt a traditional, largely subject-based approach to medical education. Within these traditional styles, they use a variety of methods, although lectures are still common.

- ✔ Peninsula, Liverpool, Manchester, Glasgow, Keele and to some extent Hull York use an extremely PBL-centred teaching method model (which we describe in the preceding section), within an integrated style.

- ✔ The rest of the UK's medical schools follow an integrated style and employ a variety of methods.

Think carefully about what environment suits you best because they're very different to one another. It's not just about what you're going to enjoy, but also about how you think and how you learn.

If you like the idea of learning through semi-guided exploration of somewhat linked topics, the PBL method may be for you. If you feel confident that seeing patients from the start of your training can motivate rather than distract, but you also like the idea of a structured learning environment, perhaps a more typical integrated course would suit you better. If you prefer a structured learning environment, with a separation of subjects into different scientific disciplines or you have research aspirations, you're most likely to thrive on a traditional course.

We can't tell you which medical school's teaching is the best; they're all good. If we were choosing for ourselves, we'd choose on the basis of our own, personal learning style. And that's exactly what you need to do.

Thinking about other differences

Medical schools differ not only in teaching styles and methods, but also in respect to whether they offer intercalated degrees or require interviews and extra exams.

Intercalating degrees

Some medical schools require or encourage you to insert a second degree alongside your primary medical qualification at the cost of spending an extra year at university between your pre-clinical and clinical years. This *intercalated degree* is generally a Bachelor of Science (BSc), though the situation is different at Oxford and Cambridge, as we explain in the later section on 'Aiming at Oxbridge'.

Cambridge, Imperial, Oxford, St Andrews and UCL include an intercalated degree as a mandatory part of their training. Most other medical schools offer intercalation as an option, either at their institution or elsewhere. The exact way in which these optional programmes are implemented varies between medical schools and changes frequently, so check with each school before applying.

If you enjoy pure science, an intercalated degree provides the opportunity to indulge in deeper study and gain experience of research methods. If you're thinking about academic medicine as a career, an intercalated degree is a good 'taster' of that experience. If you're really keen on this route, you can even customise programmes to allow further study up to MA or PhD level.

You don't have to pursue a science subject for your intercalated degree, although a big majority of students do. Some medical schools offer a wider range of programmes, including humanities, languages and social sciences.

An intercalated degree is often paced more slowly than pre-clinical or clinical work, offering a chance for medical students to experience a more typical student life. The experience can even feel like a much-appreciated holiday by comparison.

Jumping the exam hurdles

Most medical schools demand that you sit selection tests. Table 2-1 tells you which medical schools want extra exams and Table 2-2 explains the course codes.

From August 2013, Peninsula College of Medicine and Dentistry splits into two new medical schools: University of Exeter Medical School, and Plymouth University Peninsula Schools of Medicine and Dentistry. Applicants for the 2013 entry cycle onwards will be able to select either or both of these schools. Both will have similar entry criteria to the current Peninsula requirements listed in Table 2-1.

Table 2-1   Medical School Courses with Extra Exams

University	UKCAT	BMAT	GAMSAT
Aberdeen	A100		
Barts and The London School of Medicine and Dentistry	A100, A101		
Brighton and Sussex Medical School	A100		
Cambridge		A100, A101 (not compulsory)	
Cardiff	A100, A104		
Dundee	A100, A104		
Durham	A100		
East Anglia	A100, A104		
Edinburgh	A100		
Glasgow	A100		
Hull York Medical School	A100		
Keele	A100, A104		
King's College London	A100, A101, A102		
Imperial College London	A101	A100	
Leeds	A100		
Leicester	A100, A101		
Manchester	A104, A106		

(continued)

Table 2-1 *(continued)*

University	UKCAT	BMAT	GAMSAT
Newcastle	A100, A101		
Nottingham	A100, A108		A101
Oxford		A100, A101	
Peninsula College of Medicine and Dentistry	A100		A100 (if not a direct school-leaver)
Queen's University Belfast	A100		
Sheffield	A100, A104		
Southampton	A100, A101, A102		
St Andrews	A100, A990, B900		
St George's, University of London	A100		A101
Swansea			A101
University College London		A100	
Warwick University Graduate Entry	A101		

Table 2-2   UCAS Course Codes

UCAS code	Course
A100	Medicine
A101	Medicine (graduate entry 4-year programmes everywhere, except King's Extended Medical Degree)

UCAS code	Course
A102	Medicine (widening access 6-year programme at Southampton; graduate professional entry 4-year programme at King's)
A104	Medicine (including initial pre-medical/ foundation year)
A108	Medicine (including foundation year, Nottingham only)
A990	North American Medical Programme (St Andrews only)
B900	International Foundation for Medicine (St Andrews only, 1-year programme)

Applying only to medical schools without extra exams is very unwise. A much better strategy is to choose medical schools you want to study at and then figure out whether you meet their entry requirements. If that means sitting an extra exam, then so be it.

We advocate this approach, even though it means more work. The truth of the matter is, if you're really serious about medical school, you're probably going to do well in any selection test. In the long run, you're going to be happiest at a university you want to attend, not one that you thought would be easiest to get into.

The same logic applies to the folly of deciding to apply only to the medical schools that don't generally interview undergraduate candidates (Edinburgh and Southampton) because you think you won't perform well in an interview setting. You're going to face many job interviews over a career in medicine, not to mention oral exams and other tests of communication skills. Medicine isn't a profession for those unable to talk to others under pressure, so you might as well get used to it from early on.

Aiming at Oxbridge

Oxford and Cambridge are internationally prestigious ancient institutions. They have unique traditions and retain a certain glamour that other medical schools don't possess. Competition for places is exceptionally fierce because they attract the very best applicants. In this section we help demystify these two universities.

A brief history of Oxbridge

When these universities were founded in the early Middle Ages, centres of learning were almost always religious institutions; the Church was one of the few ways a person could get an education and monastic halls were the first academic houses in Oxford. They provided accommodation and structure for undergraduate life in an attempt to bring order to the chaos of hundreds of students living independently across the city.

Colleges were originally for graduate students only. They had generous endowments and permanent teaching staff. By the fourteenth century, they accepted fee-paying undergraduates and this gradually led to colleges superseding the monastic halls. Oxford's oldest colleges (University, Balliol and Merton) were established between 1249 and 1264, although no one knows which is the very oldest.

The founding date of the wider university is also uncertain but some evidence suggests that the first teaching dates back to 1096. The university grew rapidly after Henry II banned English students from attending the University of Paris in 1167.

In 1209, following a series of violent riots between Oxford's students and townsfolk, some academics fled northeast to found the University of Cambridge.

Living in colleges

Oxford and Cambridge (collectively often referred to as Oxbridge) operate *collegiate* systems, which means that each university consists of a number of more or less autonomous colleges.

The collegiate system operates similarly in both universities. Colleges are self-governing bodies under the umbrella of the broader university. The core elements of a college are a chapel, dining hall, library and student accommodation. Buildings are typically arranged around quads, sometimes of a cloistered design echoing the religious origins of the colleges. Each college has its own faculty but students are also taught by staff from other colleges; this practice is routine in medicine.

Living and studying in a college has the benefit of meeting people working across many disciplines. This arrangement can lead to a more enriching social and educational environment than being surrounded solely by medics. It broadens the mind; a useful trait in both medicine and life.

Students typically spend at least some of their years living in college accommodation, although some live out of college for differing periods of time. Medical students tend to spend a greater proportion of their time living out, largely due to the natural tendency to drift out of college accommodation over time.

Studying in tutorials

The relatively small number of students at each college combined with large permanent faculties results in excellent staff-to-student ratios. This permits the Oxbridge tutorial method of education.

Tutorials are a form of small group teaching where typically 2–4 students meet with one of the fellows attached to the college faculty to discuss a topic. Medical students typically have a few tutorials every week, on subjects paralleling whatever their lecture course is covering at the same time. They prepare short essays around relevant topics and discuss them as a group at tutorials.

This approach does involve some extra work but essay writing isn't overly onerous and you adapt to it after the first few weeks. The opportunity to discuss topics with sometimes very impressive people working in the field is definitely worth it.

Overcoming preconceptions

Students are often intimidated by the prospect of applying to Oxbridge. They may feel that the application process is too hard and that they won't make the grade. Or they may have an image of Oxbridge as old-fashioned, stuffy and elitist.

The peculiar case of the Oxbridge MA

All medical students at Oxford and Cambridge do an intercalated degree (see the earlier section 'Intercalating degrees' for more info). For historical reasons the degree awarded is a BA rather than a BSc. A holder of an Oxbridge BA may upgrade to a Master of Arts (MA) a certain number of years from starting university, on payment of a small fee and without extra study or exams.

Historically, this was to enable Oxbridge graduates to teach, as only MA holders were allowed to do so. A more whimsical (if untrue) explanation is that Oxbridge considered its education to be of such a high quality that it took some extra years for students to come to terms with all its nuances, by which time they were wise enough to receive an MA!

Only in the nineteenth century did MA degrees begin to be associated with a further level of education. Confusingly, Oxford and Cambridge also award more typical MA degrees to reward postgraduate study.

Oxbridge is elitist, but it's a 'good elitism' in the sense that it rewards nothing but high performance. Regardless of your upbringing or background, if you have talent Oxbridge recognises and rewards it. Opportunities to express that talent are almost unlimited, both in terms of study and extracurricular pursuits. Although Oxford and Cambridge do have ancient traditions, the atmosphere is far from stuffy. In fact they're very dynamic institutions, keen to stretch their students and make their time at university as rewarding as possible. At the same time, they recognise that university can be challenging and the college system allows for plenty of student welfare and support.

And don't forget, those generous college endowments mean lots of bursaries and prizes to subsidise the cost of medical school.

Oxford and Cambridge are wonderful places to live and work; don't miss out on a chance to be there because of unfounded worries. If you have the academic background to make Oxbridge a realistic prospect but are fearful of applying because of your preconceptions, strongly consider biting the bullet and going for it. Visit on open days, walk around the colleges, talk to current students. Do not feel intimidated by closed doors and college porters. If you have the talent, give Oxbridge a go!

Applying to Oxbridge

If you want to study medicine at Oxford or Cambridge, you're going to be up against the best students in the country, if not the world. The application process also has some extra steps.

First, you're going to have to choose between the two universities: you can't apply to both. Being objective about the differences between the two is almost impossible (especially because one of us went to Oxford, and is naturally slightly biased in its favour!). But it's probably fair to say that Oxford has more of a bustling feel compared to Cambridge's quieter market town atmosphere. More controversially, Cambridge may be said to possess the marginally more demanding pre-clinical programme, though both are tough.

The second key aspect is deciding whether to apply to specific colleges or to submit an 'open' application where you're randomly allocated to colleges.

We advise picking a specific college because, at the very least, it demonstrates that you have an active interest in your application and that you researched the various options. It also gives you the opportunity to explain your choice to the college at interview.

Choosing a college can be difficult: they all tend to be beautiful and superficially similar places. However, one difference is the size of the college. Large colleges have more students and can be a little more anonymous. Smaller colleges frequently have tighter knit student bodies. Some larger colleges have more generous endowments and that wealth can influence what bursaries and prizes are available, as well as the quality of student meals and accommodation. On balance, we recommend choosing a college based on personality fit rather than on architectural or financial standing.

Graduate medical applicants at Oxford and Cambridge need to complete university-specific supplementary application forms in addition to the standard application. You can find these forms at www.medsci.ox.ac.uk/study/medicine/accelerated/application-procedure and www.study.cam.ac.uk/undergraduate/courses/medicine/.

Funding Your Place

University can be expensive, particularly medicine because it lasts longer than most other courses. One consolation is that you'll probably be earning more than most other graduates, which makes up for the high initial costs.

Medical schools recognise that the cost of education is growing and all offer some bursaries, prizes and other awards in mitigation. What's on offer varies between universities, but Oxford and Cambridge have the most generous schemes available.

The NHS offers medical students substantial bursaries if you meet its criteria. Check out www.nhsbsa.nhs.uk/students for details.

Understanding the changing tuition fees

You may read a lot of scary misinformation about the changes to tuition fees starting in 2012. Here are the facts:

- Medical schools charge £9,000 per annum. The amount is reduced for poorer students through the provision of bursaries.

- From your fifth year, the NHS Student Bursary Scheme covers your tuition fees. At this stage, you're also eligible for means-tested NHS bursaries to cover maintenance costs and a reduced maintenance loan from the Student Loans Company's Student Finance England subsidiary.

✔ You pay nothing upfront. For new undergraduates, Student Loan Company loans automatically pay your tuition fees. Here's more info about the loans:

- You can opt not to take the loans, in which case you're responsible for paying your own fees.

- You can repay loans early if you want to.

- You only start repaying loans from the April after graduation at the earliest, no matter how long your course.

- Loans are repaid through the income tax system; repayments appear on your salary slip, reducing your post-tax income.

- The amount you repay per month depends solely on your income (9 per cent of the part of your pre-tax salary above £21,000 per annum), not on the amount you borrow. That threshold is index-linked and so rises over time to account for inflation.

- Interest is charged on your loan, with an index-linked element. The precise rate depends on your income, but is generally 3 per cent above the rate of inflation for most doctors after their first few years in practice.

- You stop repayments when you've repaid the loan (plus interest) or after 30 years, whichever comes first.

The mathematically astute may spot that this new system means that monthly repayments are lower than the previous regime, but that you owe a larger pot of money and that the total amount repayable is significantly greater.

A quirk of the system is that many non-medical students may never repay the full amount of their loans because of the 30-year time limit. Only those earning relatively large amounts early in their careers will end up repaying everything plus interest and most doctors will fall within this group.

Further number crunching reveals that overpaying when you start earning a higher salary (about £41,000 in today's money) may be worthwhile to whittle down the capital on which you're being charged interest.

If you're lucky enough not to need the loans, the choice of whether to take them or not depends on whether you (or your parents) can invest the money and generate a higher rate of return than the interest charged on the loan.

Whether or not to take loans and whether to repay them early are clearly very individual decisions. The above does not constitute financial advice, but merely an attempt to refute some of the frightening and frankly misleading debt stories being circulated.

The fairest summary is that medicine is still an affordable degree, but you end up repaying more over time. You still get a highly subsidised education but not quite as highly subsidised as under the old system.

Charging in the devolved administrations

Education is a devolved power in the UK and so Scotland, Wales and Northern Ireland set their own policies on tuition fees. The current situation in the devolved administrations is as follows:

- ✔ **Scotland:** Scottish students continue to pay no tuition fees. English and Northern Irish students studying in Scotland pay up to £9,000 per year. Welsh students receive support from the Welsh government.

- ✔ **Northern Ireland:** Northern Ireland students studying in Northern Ireland pay a fixed price of £3,465 in 2012/13. Those from England or Scotland are charged up to £9,000 per year, while Welsh students receive support from the Welsh government.

- ✔ **Wales:** Tuition fees at Welsh universities follow the English pattern. However, the Welsh government covers the increase for Welsh resident students, and so they don't have to pay any more than the current cost plus inflation (£3,465 in 2012). English, Scottish and Northern Irish students pay the full amount.

Paying as a graduate medical student

The arrangements for graduate medical students on five-year undergraduate medical school courses are less generous than for school-leavers. In the first four years, they're not eligible for a loan, either for tuition fees or a maintenance grant.

However, students may apply for a means-tested maintenance loan from Student Finance England and from year five they receive the same support as undergraduates.

Graduate students on accelerated fast-track courses are eligible to apply for student loans to cover the cost of their tuition fee and maintenance in their first year. In subsequent years, the NHS Bursary Scheme pays £3,375 of each year's tuition fee. Students are eligible to apply for a student loan to fund the £5,625 shortfall.

Graduate medical students domiciled in England and Wales can also apply for means-tested maintenance loans from the NHS Student Bursaries Unit.

Chapter 3

Planning Your Application

. . . .

In This Chapter

▶ Knowing when to apply

▶ Grasping how medical school applications work

▶ Discussing different routes into medical school

. . . .

*T*o get into medical school you need to complete and submit an application. It's your opportunity to make a great first impression. A strong application puts you in pole position for this most competitive of races.

All the UK's medical schools accept applications only through the Universities and Colleges Admissions Service (UCAS). UCAS acts as a portal to submit your application, monitor its progress and manage your offers.

In this chapter we cover how UCAS works, lead you through completing the application form and also discuss how to apply to medical school if you're not a typical school-leaver or if you're applying from outside the UK.

Timing Your Application

University applications make for a hectic final two years of school. You can feel as if you're trying to keep several balls in the air at the same time: deciding what subject you want to do and where you want to study, and maintaining your existing obligations and dealing with academic pressures, not to mention finding time to relax and have a life.

If you're applying to medical school, you also need to fit in work experience and extra selection tests. Our flowchart (Figure 3-1) will help you organise your time during this fast-paced period.

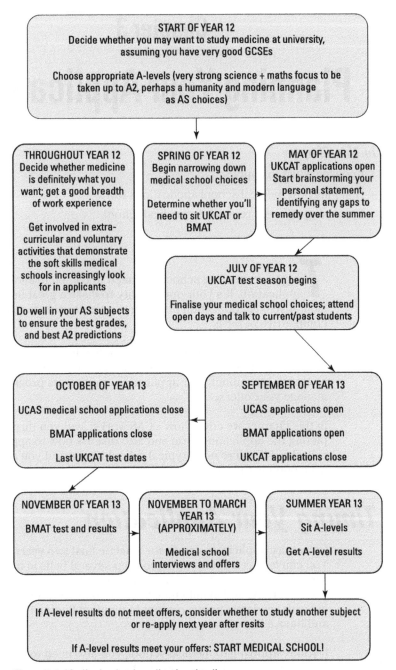

Figure 3-1: Medical school application timeline.

Medical students need to finalise and submit their application by mid-October at the latest (15 October in a typical year). This time-frame is significantly earlier than for other university applicants. Although seeing your friends happily forgetting about university applications while you're mired in the details of your UCAS form can be annoying, the earlier date is necessary because of the drawn-out nature of medical school applications.

 If you're a graduate applicant to Oxford or Cambridge Universities (Oxbridge), don't forget to submit your university-specific graduate application forms by this date too (check out the later section 'Applying as a graduate' for more information).

Using UCAS

UCAS operates a computerised university application system. Fortunately, the process is straightforward and user-friendly and the website (at www.ucas.ac.uk) generally works very well.

To begin an application, go to the website. Click Apply and follow the on-screen instructions. You're prompted to register a user-name and password and are then directed to the secure online application form. The registration process is a breeze for today's computer-literate generation.

When you're registered with UCAS, you can begin completing your application form. You can save a partially completed form, but remember not to submit it until you've finished completely.

The UCAS form has several sections:

- ✔ **Personal details:** Typical administrative content such as your name and address.

- ✔ **Additional information:** UK applicants provide information on ethnic origin and can choose to supply details about parental and occupational background.

  More importantly, you also have an opportunity to list any courses or activities that you've done to prepare for higher education. For example, Medsim (www.workshop-uk.net/medsim) offers simulations of clinical scenarios, while our Get into Medical School website (www.getintomedicalschool.org) offers courses on UKCAT, BMAT and interview skills. University open days don't count as eligible activities for this section.

✔ **Student finance:** Only UK applicants see this section and it's customised to your part of the country. It allows UCAS to communicate with the Student Loans Company (Student Awards Agency in Scotland) to streamline your loan applications.

✔ **Choices:** You can apply to up to five institutions but only four medical schools. If you definitely don't want to study anything else and prefer to reapply if you don't get in this year, leave the fifth choice blank. Undergraduates cannot apply to both Oxford and Cambridge.

If you don't mind doing a different degree, you can put down another course. But regardless, we strongly advise you to tailor your personal statement very directly to medicine.

Your choices are *not* ranked by preference, and universities do *not* see what other institutions you're applying to.

✔ **Education:** You have to enter all qualifications, including ones for which you have yet to sit the final exam. Entering module marks is optional: if they're good, we advise you to enter them.

If you have done poorly in a particular module you can opt not to include it, but this may raise unwelcome questions in shortlisters' minds and at interviews. The better option can be to include it and then explain how you're remedying it in your personal statement.

✔ **Employment:** This refers to paid employment, but includes part-time jobs and temporary positions. Include everything because doing so is a great way to demonstrate to medical schools that you're an experienced, reliable, punctual, hardworking team player.

✔ **Your personal statement:** This section of the form is absolutely crucial and can make a real difference to your chances of getting into medical school. In fact it's so important that we dedicate the whole of Chapter 5 to it.

✔ **Your reference:** If you're applying through a school or college, you don't fill out this section; instead the institution supplies your reference for you.

If you're applying independently, you can supply details of a referee. Remember to pick someone in a position of authority who you can implicitly trust to give you a good reference (we talk more about references in Chapter 4).

The role of contextual data

From the 2012 cycle onwards, UCAS provides universities with contextual information about you in the form of data about your school's socio-economic make-up and academic performance. Universities can choose to use this information to identify students with raw talent who are significantly outperforming in spite of unfavourable circumstances. For example, they can compare your results to those of others from a similar background to see if you're doing a lot better than might be expected. They can then use this data to select candidates for interviews or offers who would otherwise not have been short-listed.

Some medical schools do use the data in this way, but the intense competition means that they have only a little leeway. Although the contextual information can make a difference, we advise you not to rely on it: getting top grades is always preferable.

After completing all the sections, click View All Details to review your application and make sure that it's correct. Then agree with the Declaration, which essentially confirms that everything you've written is the truth, and move on to Pay and Send. If you're applying through a school or college, it arranges payment on your behalf, although depending on the institution you may have to reimburse it at a later date. Otherwise, you pay UCAS directly using a credit or debit card (alternative methods are available if you contact the Customer Service Unit on 0871 4680468).

After you submit your application, UCAS sends you a welcome letter confirming your details and choices. It allows your chosen medical schools to view your application, and they decide whether to shortlist you for an interview.

As you go through the rest of the application cycle, UCAS informs you of your progress by regular letters. You can receive these by normal mail or electronically by logging in through the Track progress link on the UCAS home page.

Taking a Different Path

Not everyone applies to medical school directly after their A-levels. Some people do another degree first, others decide to go into medicine after working in a different field and some apply from abroad.

Applying as a graduate

An increasing number of graduates want to study medicine. Traditionally, there was only one way to do this: graduates had to apply for the full undergraduate programme. Nowadays graduates face a choice. They can still opt to apply for the undergraduate courses, but they can also choose to apply for accelerated 'fast-track' graduate-entry medicine courses instead. Accelerated courses are typically a year shorter than undergraduate courses, and are correspondingly more intensive.

Graduates frequently ask us which route offers the best odds of getting into medical school. Our answer is that both are challenging:

- ✔ **Accelerated courses:** These are highly competitive because your fellow candidates are extremely motivated and driven, perhaps more so than school-leavers applying to undergraduate courses.

- ✔ **Undergraduate courses:** You can avoid this extra competition by applying for the full undergraduate course, but you then have to justify to medical schools why you've opted against the accelerated course. Some reasonable explanations exist, for example, not having a science-based first degree or it being a long time since you studied the sciences, but even this can be a very hard sell.

Getting into medical school is going to be difficult with either route, so if you're eligible for both options you might as well apply for the accelerated courses. This advice is especially sound if you're keen to be doctoring (and earning!) as soon as possible.

Of course, graduates who don't meet the entry requirements for accelerated programmes can apply for a full-length undergraduate course, provided they meet the relevant entry criteria.

Table 3-1 lists the medical schools offering a fast-track course alongside its entry requirements. Keele University isn't listed because, as of 2012, it no longer accepts new entrants to its fast-track course.

Table 3-1 Fast-Track Graduate-Entry Medical Schools

Medical School	1st Degree Entry Requirements	Selection Test Required	A-levels if 1st Degree Not Science-Based
Barts and The London	2:1	UKCAT	BB Biology and Chemistry
Birmingham	1st preferred	None	BBB inc. Chemistry as bare minimum
Bristol	2:1	None	BBB inc. two sciences
Cambridge	1st preferred, 2:1 minimum	BMAT optional	Must have Chemistry
Imperial	2:1 (or PhD)	UKCAT	Must have science-based degree
King's College London	2:1 (or further degree with merit)	UKCAT	Not specified
Leicester	2:1 (and have been working full-time and paid in caring role)	UKCAT	Not specified
Liverpool	2:1	None	Not specified
Newcastle	2:1 (or qualified healthcare profes-sional)	UKCAT	Not specified
Nottingham	2:2	GAMSAT	Not specified but extensive healthcare work experi-ence is neces-sary
Oxford	2:1 (1st preferred)	BMAT	Must have science-based degree *and* 2 science A-levels

(continued)

Table 3-1 (continued)

Medical School	1st Degree Entry Requirements	Selection Test Required	A-levels if 1st Degree Not Science-Based
Southampton	2:1	UKCAT	A-level Chemistry
St George's, University of London	2:2	GAMSAT	Not specified
Swansea	2:1	GAMSAT	Biology or Chemistry
Warwick	2:1 (or 2:2 with PhD)	UKCAT	Not specified

Assessing application options without science A-levels

You can become a doctor without science A-levels; if you're also a graduate you may even be able to apply for a fast-track course (check out the preceding section for more information on that route). This section focuses on routes into medicine if you don't meet the criteria for accelerated graduate-entry medicine.

Medical schools increasingly recognise that not everyone follows the same route through life. People who have the potential to be good doctors may not have science A-levels and so not meet the usual entry criteria for undergraduate medicine. Some medical schools allow you to acquire this scientific knowledge and related practical skills by studying for an extra year prior to starting medical school proper. These programmes are sometimes called *foundation courses*.

Some of these courses also attempt to widen access to medicine by offering a relatively higher percentage of contextual offers than for the typical course. Contextual offers are slightly reduced requirements, made on the basis of evidence of a disadvantaged educational and/or home background. Universities use publicly available data (often from UCAS) about your school to determine whether a contextual offer is appropriate, although they can draw on other written evidence as well. Check out the earlier sidebar 'The role of contextual data' for more on this subject.

If you're accepted onto one of these courses and successfully complete it, you're typically offered an automatic place at medical school.

Application is restricted to those who don't meet the standard course entry requirements. So this isn't a backdoor route into medical school for those already eligible for direct entry!

Table 3-2 has information on foundation courses and their entry requirements. Research them carefully to ensure that you meet their detailed entry requirements.

Table 3-2   Medical Schools with Foundation Courses

Medical School	A-level Entry Requirements
Bristol	AAA/A*AB with 1 or 0 sciences
	Or 2:2 non-science degree plus BBB/ABC non-science A-levels
	Bristol do not technically define this as a foundation course, and it will be discontinued from 2014
Cardiff	AAA with 1 or 0 sciences
Dundee	AAA with 1 or 0 sciences
	AAAAB Scottish Highers with 1 or 0 sciences
Durham	The Foundation Programme is open to those without A-levels
East Anglia (Norwich Medical School)	BBB with 1 or 0 sciences
	Contextual requirements apply
Keele	4 A levels or AAA/A*AB plus B at AS level with no Chemistry
	Or 2:1 graduate degree without science A-levels
King's College London	Contextual offer based on A-levels & 1 AS level *including* Chemistry and Biology with BBB as a minimum; technically the KCL 6-year course is a slowed-down standard medical degree for those educated non-selectively (outside of the comprehensive system), and is *not* a true foundation course

(continued)

Table 3-2 (continued)

Medical School	A-level Entry Requirements
Leeds (via University of Bradford course)	CC
Liverpool	Apply directly to school, not via UCAS; no A-levels required
Manchester	AAB with no Chemistry
Sheffield	AAA with no science subjects
Southampton	BCC *including* Chemistry and Biology. Contextual factors considered
St George's, University of London	No A-levels required; course 'designed for' mature students

In addition, there are also standalone Access to Medicine diplomas. These don't guarantee a place at medical school, but many medical schools do see them as evidence of equivalence to a science A-level background.

These courses are intended for students with either non-science A-levels at lower grades than would be suitable for the courses in Table 3-2, or without A-levels at all.

If you choose this route, you need subsequently to apply to medical school as an undergraduate. The level of competition is such that you usually have to pass the Access course with distinction to stand a realistic chance of getting in.

Not all medical schools view Access to Medicine diplomas as being a sufficient qualification and some require you to sit extra selection tests, such as the UKCAT or the GAMSAT, as part of your application. More detailed information on how specific medical schools treat Access to Medicine diplomas can be found on individual school websites. However, enough medical schools do accept them (with or without additional tests) to give you a broad choice of potential universities to apply to on completion of the diploma.

Table 3-3 lists colleges that offer these courses, the precise name of the course and the college website address for further information.

Table 3-3   Standalone Access to Medicine Courses

Further Education College	Access to Medicine Course Title	College Website Address
City and Islington College	Access to Medicine and Medical Biosciences	www.candi.ac.uk
Lambeth College	Medicine and Dentistry (Medical and Biomedical Science) – OCNLR Access to Higher Education	www.lambethcollege.ac.uk
Liverpool Community College	The Access Programme: Science & Technology Pathway	www.liv-coll.ac.uk
The Manchester College	Medicine	www.themanchester college.ac.uk
Stafford College	Access to HE Diploma (Medicine and Health Professions)	www.staffordcoll.ac.uk
Sussex Downs Adult College	Access to Medicine	www.sussexdowns.ac.uk
The College of West Anglia	Access to Medicine and Dentistry	www.cwa.ac.uk

Considering applications from outside the UK

The UK has a long history of welcoming students from all parts of the world, and overseas candidates continue to be most welcome at UK medical schools.

If you're a European Union (EU) applicant, EU legislation theoretically places you on an equal footing with UK applicants. You still need to demonstrate a high level of fluency in English and meet equivalent entry requirements to UK applicants, but you can otherwise apply as normal. Chapter 4 has more details on International Baccalaureate and European Baccalaureate requirements.

UK medical schools can accept students from outside of the EU, but these cannot represent more than 7.5 per cent of their total combined intake. Individual medical schools are more restrictive and some require applicants to come from countries without universities offering primary medical degrees. The precise requirements change frequently, so you're best advised to ask individual medical schools about their policy towards non-EU students.

All non-native English speakers must take the International English Language Testing System (IELTS) Academic Test. The test comprises four modules – listening, reading, writing and speaking – and is 2 hours and 45 minutes long in total. The listening, reading and writing components are completed in one sitting. The speaking component may be taken up to seven days before or after the other tests, depending on the test centre.

For a set fee, you can take the test in over 500 locations worldwide (more information at www.ielts.org).

International medical students pay full tuition fees. These vary between medical schools, but are much higher than domestic rates. Typical rates are in the region of £25,000 per year, such that a full medical degree might cost over £125,000 in fees alone. Living costs in the UK are also high, and higher still in London.

You need to get a student immigration visa to enter the UK and can't claim welfare or benefits; in addition, strict limits apply to what kinds of paid work you can undertake while studying here. The United Kingdom Border Agency manages immigration issues; you can find more information about visas on their website (www.ukba.homeoffice.gov.uk).

In addition, the UK Council for International Student Affairs (www.ukcisa.org.uk) has a wealth of further, more general information about studying in the UK.

Chapter 4

Building Your Foundation for Medical School

*N*o one simply walks into medical school: you need to prove that you deserve a place.

Medical schools want candidates with excellent academic records who have realistic views of medicine. They need people who are mature enough to know their own strengths and limitations, and who are willing to work hard.

All this means that you need to have achieved excellent grades so far, have top predictions for future exams and have enough work experience to convince medical schools (and yourself) that medicine is the right career for you.

In this chapter we cover all these areas in detail. We also explain why universities are interested in your non-academic activities and give you tips on getting a good reference. And because you're busy, we show you how to maximise the time to your application deadline.

Getting the Necessary Grades

Only those with strong academic records get into medical school. You need excellent GCSE results, strong results in AS exams and equally good predictions for A2 grades. Competition is very stiff and universities have a hard time choosing between candidates with equally sterling academic records.

To help separate the good from the great, most medical schools use extra exams such as the United Kingdom Clinical Aptitude Test (UKCAT) or the Bio-Medical Admissions Test (BMAT). For graduate entry, some medical schools require the Graduate Australian Medical School Admissions Test (GAMSAT). We discuss the UKCAT in much more detail in Chapters 6 and 7, the BMAT in Chapters 8 and 9 and the GAMSAT in Chapter 10.

Because you're applying to four medical schools, you'll probably need to sit at least one extra exam, usually the UKCAT. However, candidates applying to Oxbridge, Imperial and UCL also need to sit the BMAT.

Multiple extra tests taken in quick succession are stressful. Plan your revision schedule and exam dates in advance so that you have time to focus on each test in turn.

Counting up your GSCEs

Table 4-1 contains the detailed GCSE requirements of each medical school.

Although you need to be aware of these minimum requirements before applying, in practice studying them in detail isn't helpful. Most of your competition hasn't simply met a minimum level of competency. They're straight A/A* students or only slightly off that impeccable standard. To succeed against such top-level candidates, you need to match or exceed them.

For universities that require extra tests, a good UKCAT or BMAT score can partially compensate for a slightly below-par GCSE or AS performance. It can't make up for a poor record, but it can make a difference in borderline cases.

Table 4-1	GCSE Requirements for Medicine			
Medical School	**Sciences**	**Maths**	**English**	**Restrictions**
Aberdeen	Recommended	C	C	
Barts and The London	BB	B	B	AAABBB minimum
Birmingham	A	A	A	7+ A* typically A*s in English, maths and all sciences

Medical School	Sciences	Maths	English	Restrictions
Brighton and Sussex		B	B	
Bristol	AA	A	A	5+ A/A*
Cambridge	CC	C		
Cardiff	AA/AAB	B	B	5+ A* typical
Dundee	Biology			
Durham	CC/CCC	C	C	5+ C
East Anglia	AA/AAA	A	A	6+ A
Edinburgh	BB	B	B	6+ A* typical
Glasgow	Biology B		B	
Hull York		A	A	6+ A–C
Imperial	BBB	B	B	
Keele	BB/BBB	B	B	4+ A
King's College London		B	B	
Lancaster				Not specified
Leeds	BB/BBB	B	B	6+ B
Leicester	CC	C	C	Higher grades score higher
Liverpool	BB	B	B	9+ C
Manchester	BB	B	B	5+ A
Newcastle	Biology and Chemistry A if not A2/AS			
Nottingham	AA/AAA	B	B	6+ A
Oxford	Biology and Physics A if not at A2	A if not at A2		9+ A* typical successful applicant
Peninsula	CC	C	C	7+ C

(continued)

Table 4-1 *(continued)*

Medical School	Sciences	Maths	English	Restrictions
Queen's Belfast				9+ B
Sheffield	CC/CCC	C	C	6+ A
Southampton	BB/BBB	B	B	7+ B
St Andrew's	B if not A2/AS	B if not A2/AS	B if not A2/AS	
St George's		B		8+ A average
University College London		B	B	Foreign Language C

Notching up A-levels

Table 4-2 contains information on the A-level entry requirements at each medical school.

If a specific AS-level grade is also demanded, we note this in lower case in the A-level Grades or Restrictions columns. The Restrictions column tells you whether the university requires specific subject combinations from Chemistry (C), Biology (B), Maths (M) or Physics (P).

Table 4-2   A-level Requirements for Medicine

Medical School	A-level Grades	Restrictions
Aberdeen	AAA	C and 1+ of B/M/P
Barts and The London	AAAb	2+ sciences, B or C at least to grade b at AS-level
Birmingham	AAA	B and C and 1+ of M/P
Brighton and Sussex	AAA (3rd grade can be B if you gain an A* or C if 2A*)	C + B to grade A
Bristol	AAA	C and 1+ of B/P

Medical School	A-level Grades	Restrictions
Cambridge	A*AA	Typically C and 2+ of B/P/M. Does vary slightly by college
Cardiff	AAAc	2+ sciences, with B or C at least to grade b at AS-level
Dundee	AAA	C and 1+ of B/P
Durham	AAA	1+ of C/B
East Anglia	AAA	B
Edinburgh	AAAb	C and 1+ of B/P/M
Glasgow	AAA	C and 1+ of B/P/M
Hull York	AAAb	C + B
Imperial	AAAb	2+ sciences, C or B at least to grade b at AS-level
Keele	AAA (3rd grade can be B if you gain an A*)	1+ of C/B and 1+ of P/M
King's College London	AAAb/AAaab	1+ C/B at A2; other at AS if not at A2
Lancaster	AAAb	C + B
Leeds	AAA	C
Leicester	AAA	C + B
Liverpool	AAAb	C + B
Manchester	AAA	C and 1+ of B/P/M
Newcastle	AAA	1+ of C/B
Nottingham	AAA	C + B
Oxford	A*AA	C and 1+ of B/P/M
Peninsula	A*AA/AAAc	C + B (at least to AS)
Queen's Belfast	AAAa	C and 1+ of B/P/M
Sheffield	AAA (abbb expected at AS)	C + 1+ of B/P

(continued)

Table 4-2 (continued)

Medical School	A-level Grades	Restrictions
Southampton	AAA	1+ C/B at A2; other at AS if not at A2
St Andrew's	AAA	C and 1+ of B/P/M
St George's	AAAb	1+ C/B at A2; other at AS if not at A2
University College London	AAA plus 4th subject AS pass	C + B; contrasting 3rd subject preferred

Do check that you have the subject combinations and grade predictions required by your chosen medical schools, but bear in mind that there is a difference between the minimum grades that a university requires from successful applicants and the grades that a typical successful applicant actually achieves. The latter is a better indicator of your chances, even if universities generally only publish the former.

The most versatile A2 combination for medical school applications is Chemistry and Biology alongside at least one of Maths and Physics, with predictions of at least AAA. A fourth A2 grade A is helpful and the more A*s the better.

If your dilemma is between taking four A-levels or the standard 3, getting A*AA is more impressive than AAAA but A*AAA is better than both. In other words, think honestly about how good you really are and maximise the impact of your predicted grades.

You definitely need at least one A* if applying to either Oxford or Cambridge.

Medical schools can exercise flexibility with respect to offers. For example, if someone is exceptionally well suited to medicine but has a slightly poorer academic record than typical (and has a valid justification for this), a medical school may lower its typical offer requirements slightly. Nonetheless, don't rely on medical schools making such contextual offers to gain a place; in the face of extreme competition, stronger grades have a natural tendency to trump contextual factors.

Two more A-levels to consider

General studies and critical thinking A-levels are great for deepening the way you approach studying and for understanding the basis of academic thought. Unfortunately, they don't typically contribute to medical school requirements (although a few universities do consider them). You can check the latest prospectuses for details, but to give yourself maximum flexibility you should perform well in three other A2 A-levels regardless of whether you sit these two exams as well.

Scoring with Scottish Highers and IBs

Table 4-3 lists the Scottish Highers or International Baccalaureate (IB) results that medical schools require for their undergraduate courses. Those with better predictions have significantly improved chances of getting into medical school compared to those meeting the minimum requirement.

Universities apply similar restrictions to subject choices in these exams as with A-levels (which we outline earlier in Table 4-2). Their prospectuses contain more information, but the most flexible package contains strong elements of Chemistry, Biology and Maths.

English universities tend to demand a strong Scottish Advanced Higher (AH) performance. Similarly, most focus on performance in Higher Level (HL) IB subjects, not just on the aggregate IB score.

Table 4-3	Scottish Highers and IB Requirements	
Medical School	*Scottish Highers*	*IB results*
Aberdeen	AAAAB	6/6/6 at HL
Barts and The London	AB at AH + AAA	6/6/5 at HL
Birmingham	AAA at AH + AA	6/6/6 at HL, 36 total
Brighton and Sussex	370+ UCAS points	6/6/6 at HL, 38 total
Bristol	AA at AH + AAA	6/6/6 at HL, 37 total
Cambridge	AAA at AH	7/7/6–7/7/7 at HL, 40–42 total

(continued)

Table 4-3 *(continued)*

Medical School	Scottish Highers	IB results
Cardiff	2A at AH + AAB	6/6/6 at HL, 36 total
Dundee	AAABB	6/6/6 at HL, 37 total
Durham	AAAAA	6/5/5 at HL, 38 total
East Anglia	AAA at AH + B	6/6/6 at HL, 34 total
Edinburgh	AAAAB	7/6/6 at HL, 37 total
Glasgow	AAAAB	6 at HL (Chemistry), 36 total
Hull York	AA at AH + AB	6/6/5 at HL, 36 total
Imperial	AAA at AH + BB	6/6 at Biology + Chemistry, 38 total
Keele	360+ UCAS points at AH	6/6/6 at HL, 35 total
King's College London	AA at AH + ABB	6/6/6 at HL, 38 total
Lancaster	AA at AH + AAB	6/6/6 at HL, 36 total
Leeds	AB at AH + AAA	6/6/6 at HL, 36 total
Leicester	AAA at AH	6/6/6 at HL, 36 total
Liverpool	AA at AH + AAB	6/6/6 at HL, 36 total
Manchester	AAA at AH	7/6/6 at HL, 37 total
Newcastle	AAAAA	6/5/5 at HL, 38 total
Nottingham	AAB at AH	6/6/6 at HL, 36 total
Oxford	AA at AH + AAA	7/6/6 at HL, 39 total
Peninsula	AAA at AH	6/6 at HL, 36–38 total
Queen's Belfast	Not specified	6/6/6 at HL, 36 total
Sheffield	AA at AH + AAB	6/6/6 at HL, 37 total
Southampton	AB at AH + AAA	6/6/6 at HL, 36 total
St Andrew's	AAAAB	7/6/6 at HL, 38 total
St George's	AAB at AH + AA	6/6/5 at HL
University College London	AAA at AH	6/6/5 at HL, 38 total

Of A*s and grade inflation

One of the most persistent criticisms of A-level exams is grade inflation. An influential report suggests that the same student would score at least two grades higher in 2006 than they would have in 1988. Teachers insist that this difference is the result of improved teaching, but universities are finding it more and more difficult to discriminate between students, leading to the introduction of additional tests such as the BMAT and UKCAT.

Under public pressure, the government introduced an A* grade for A2 exams, awarded only to those scoring above 90 per cent. So far, only Oxford and Cambridge absolutely insist on candidates getting at least 1 A*, but if previous trends are anything to go by, more institutions are going to demand it in years to come.

Looking at other options

Certain international exams can act as evidence of strong academic achievement. The European Baccalaureate (EB) is one such exam. EB entry requirements vary, but a typical candidate scores at least 85 per cent. Check the latest requirements with individual medical schools.

Graduate entry medicine is highly competitive. Typical entry requirements are a 2:1 grade (sometimes restricted to life sciences) and often a First. You can find more information on graduate applications, including entry requirements, in Chapter 3.

Showing Commitment to Your Chosen Career

A strong academic record is necessary but not sufficient for getting into medical school. Universities want enthusiastic students. You can demonstrate your commitment to medicine in two main ways:

- ✔ Keeping abreast with medical current affairs and being clear about their implications.
- ✔ Gaining experience in a variety of medical settings and reflecting upon it thoughtfully and insightfully.

Maintaining your interest

You can stay up to date with the latest medical news in many ways, such as by reading the health sections of major broadsheet newspapers and the websites of news agencies, or subscribing to journals such as the *Student British Medical Journal* (*Student BMJ*).

You can also set up a small discussion group with other students applying to medical school, meeting regularly to exchange interesting news stories and opinions. If you have an enthusiastic science teacher or careers adviser, you might be able to persuade them to chair and facilitate the discussions.

We run a free blog at *Get into Medicine UK* (www.getintomedicine uk.com). Subscribe to its feed to stay in touch with the latest health news. We also include key questions that put each story into its wider medical and ethical context, and can be used to spur further thought or discussion.

Experiencing healthcare first-hand

Most people know about life as a doctor from what they see on TV or from (we hope) rare visits to GP surgeries or hospitals. The training that medical schools give students is long, difficult and very expensive, so schools want to be confident that students are going to last the course. They need to know that you're familiar with what a doctor actually does and the best way to demonstrate this is through work experience.

Lots of options are available but work experience is about quality rather than quantity. The experience is most effective – and most fun – when you learn something that's going to make you a better doctor. Add variety to your placements. For example, if your experience to date consists of glamorous stints in high-profile hospitals or research centres, try balancing that out with local hospice or charity work.

Students who don't have the advantage of medical friends or family can encounter difficulty in getting work experience placements. Writing letters to healthcare organisations frequently results in polite rebuffs. A better starting point is to make a personal connection with someone working in medicine. If you can't think of anyone, try your GP. Most are glad to talk to someone interested in what they do. But don't simply turn up at the surgery asking to talk and don't just write in hoping for the best. Call up and book an appointment specifically to discuss your interest in a career in medicine.

When you're in front of the GP, explain your interest and what you've done so far, and ask for advice.

People generally love an opportunity to talk about things they know. Steer the conversation towards the topic you want to discuss (in this case, getting some work experience). This approach is far more effective than making direct requests.

Shadowing a doctor

Shadowing GPs or hospital doctors is great for discovering what a doctor does. Most hospitals usually have one or two doctors who love spending time with work experience students and showing them what the job involves. If you already have a personal contact working in healthcare, ask that person to point you in the right direction.

If you're really stuck, call your local hospital and ask to speak to the medical staffing or human resources department and talk to them about the possibility of getting some work experience in medicine. They tend to know which doctors are open to having students.

In general, we suggest using a personal contact if possible, because human resources departments can, ironically, sometimes be a bit impersonal. They may also tie you up in paperwork to clear you for clinical shadowing that isn't always absolutely necessary. But if you haven't got a contact in the system already and your GP isn't proving helpful, they're your best bet for getting work experience.

Here are some aspects to watch out for during your work experience:

- ✔ Observe the structure of a doctor's day.

- ✔ Pay attention to the different things doctors do in addition to treating patients.

- ✔ Make a note of things that make their job easier and of the hassles they face.

- ✔ Think about how they interact with patients and other health professionals.

Many students trundle through their work experience in a daze. Don't let this be you. You're not there to learn lots of complex medical information, so don't worry if some of it goes over your head. Your task is to find out what being a doctor is like so that you can demonstrate this knowledge on the UCAS personal statement and in interviews. Stay alert and make the most of the opportunity!

Working in a hospice or for a charity

In order to add balance, try helping at a local hospice or charity. This may be hard to arrange because of the time-consuming background checks sometimes required, but charities in particular are often keen to get free help.

Hospice and charity work is great for proving that you understand the gritty, emotionally stressful side of working with ill people. It also helps you develop and demonstrate good communication skills.

Getting a job in healthcare

Although getting a job in healthcare can be challenging for those under 18, if you can swing it, a stint working as a hospital porter or GP receptionist is fantastic experience. You get to see how the complex bureaucracy and different elements of the NHS mesh together in practice, and the experience tells shortlisters that you have basic life skills such as getting to work on time and working in a team.

Plus, you have the added benefit of money coming in!

NHS jobs are advertised online at www.jobs.nhs.uk, with volunteer posts listed alongside paid employment.

Demonstrating That You Have the Right Stuff

Doctors are more than walking medical textbooks. They support people during the most challenging times of their lives and they lead teams through nerve-wracking situations. Author Tom Wolfe memorably described NASA's astronauts as having 'the right stuff'. Medical schools place an equally strong emphasis on choosing people with the personality to cope with being a doctor (the *soft* skills) as they do on the ability to gain knowledge and technical ability (the *hard* skills).

Proving that you have these soft skills requires more than getting good grades and collecting work experience. The skills honed by extracurricular activities map neatly onto the technical skills needed by doctors.

Joining in at school

You probably don't realise how much you do at school. Many of the activities that schools offer outside of the classroom teach you skills that you can highlight in your application to medical school.

Table 4-4 lists some of the extracurricular activities schools frequently offer together with the personal qualities that they call upon.

Table 4-4	Extracurricular Activities at School
Activity	*Skills Demonstrated*
Sports	Team-working, leadership
Drama	Team-working, organisation, attention to detail, empathy
Combined Cadet Force and Duke of Edinburgh Awards	Leadership, team-working, communication, organisation
Debating Society	Organisation, communication
Community Service	Communication, empathy
School Governance (for example, house prefect, student council role)	Organisation, team-working, leadership
Music and the Arts	Creativity, initiative

Getting involved in your community

If your school doesn't offer many extracurricular options, think about what you can do in your local community to demonstrate your soft skills and personal qualities.

Table 4-5 lists a few options for community work and the qualities that they highlight.

Table 4-5	Community Projects
Community Project	*Skills Demonstrated*
Charitable Works	Empathy, team-working, communication, organisation
Young Enterprise Schemes	Initiative, leadership, organisation, attention to detail
Local Theatre/Music Group	Creativity, initiative, team-working, punctuality, working with the public
Part-time/weekend work	Team-working, attention to detail, organisation, punctuality, working with the public
Civic Activity (helping out with residents' associations, urban gardening/beautification projects, restoring wetlands, environmental projects and so forth)	Empathy, initiative, organisation, leadership, team-working, dedication
Personal Hobbies	Depends on the hobby but may include attention to detail, organisation, initiative and the awareness of a need to relax
Any community equivalent of the activities in Table 4-4	As per the relevant entry for the activity in Table 4-4

Reflecting on Your Progress

Reflection is the skill that you use when you think about the past and try to understand the following:

- ✔ What happened?
- ✔ Why did it happen?
- ✔ What lessons can you draw?
- ✔ How may you do things better in the future?

In short, reflection is about being an active participant in life, as opposed to clocking in and out mindlessly.

Once you've completed plenty of work experience (see the earlier section 'Showing Commitment to Your Chosen Career') and been involved in lots of activities inside and out of school (as we describe in 'Demonstrating that You Have the Right Stuff' earlier in this chapter), you need to discuss what you learned sensitively and insightfully. Medical schools are increasingly keen that students demonstrate this ability to reflect on their actions.

The great advantage of being reflective is that it makes life more efficient. For instance, if you reflect on the activities you've undertaken so far, you can identify what other activities you still need to undertake to satisfy the people doing the shortlisting. You can then use your remaining time to fill the gaps. In this way, reflection makes your life easier and more productive.

Medical schools aren't the only institutions that like thoughtful and reflective students. Medical regulators such as the General Medical Council now insist that doctors use reflective practice. Getting into the habit early is useful.

A good starting point for reflection is to grab a big sheet of blank paper and carry out the following steps:

1. **Put your name in the middle.** Now at least you have something concrete written down on that scary blank page to help focus your mind! Spend 10 minutes brainstorming around anything you do during the week that may relate to your medical school application.

2. **Scribble each activity down on the page in the area around your name.** Don't analyse each activity at this stage and don't try to organise them. Just get them all down on paper.

3. **Put the sheet away somewhere safe.** Your brain continues to think about it at an unconscious level. Over the next few days, as you go through your normal routine, you'll probably remember a few more activities. Go back to the sheet and write them down.

4. **Retrieve the paper after a couple of weeks and think about the skills demonstrated with each activity.** You can use Tables 4-1 and 4-2 from the earlier 'Getting the Necessary Grades' section as a jumping-off point, but be creative and think laterally about the personal qualities each activity demands and demonstrates. You should now have a long list of activities together with a still longer list of soft skills (which we define in the earlier section 'Demonstrating That You Have the Right Stuff').

5. **Think about the skills a doctor needs.** We talk about these skills in Chapter 1.

6. **Compare your list of personal qualities with those skills and note any glaring omissions.** In the time you have left before you submit your application, focus on taking part in extracurricular activities that patch up the gaps.

In Chapter 5, we tell you how to incorporate this information into your UCAS personal statement. And in Chapter 12, we tell you how you can use it to impress interviewers. So don't throw away that brainstormed piece of paper just yet!

Getting a Good Reference

A good reference isn't going to get you into medical school, but a bad one can certainly keep you out. If you're still at school, you probably won't have a choice of referee; one will be appointed for you. Fortunately, it's rare for a school to write a bad reference, but it's still worth making sure. Try to find out who the referee is – mostly likely a department head, the headteacher or principal, a sixth form tutor or a careers adviser – but don't pester the person about your reference. Instead, concentrate on keeping your grades up and being an active, responsible and productive member of your school.

Do let your assigned referee know that you're interested in medicine. A nice way of doing this is to ask the person for advice about your application; referees have probably seen lots of medical school candidates over the years. What you actually ask about isn't all that important; it's just a way of making contact. Even if the advice you receive is unremarkable, you've still demonstrated your interest and the referee may remember that fact when the time comes to write your reference.

If you do have a choice of referee, you're probably no longer at school. Think about where you've worked or studied. Pick someone fairly senior who knows you well and has seen you working and interacting with others.

If you've worked in a healthcare setting and got on well with your manager or a doctor in the team, ask for a reference. Such people can be ideal referees because they not only know how you work, but can also draw on their advanced understanding of what it takes to be a good doctor.

Picking someone superficially friendly may seem like the easy option, but it's wisest to pick someone you can trust not to say one thing to your face and then write something else down as your reference.

Chapter 5

Writing Your UCAS Personal Statement

*T*he medical schools considering your application have never met you and don't know you from Adam. For them, your Universities and Colleges Admissions Service (UCAS) personal statement *is* you. Unless you include all the wonderful things you have done on your UCAS form, and more specifically in your personal statement, universities won't know a thing about them.

Medical schools receive thousands of applications from hopeful students and so making sure that you stand out is essential. A good personal statement catches the eye of the people shortlisting candidates for interviews and is frequently the difference between gaining an interview and being rejected.

The good news is that with a bit of time and practice, you can create a great personal statement that catches the shortlisters' attention. In this chapter, we cover the key content that needs to be in your statement, review the basics of good writing, give you tips on how to sell yourself without coming across as forced or affected, and, perhaps most importantly, tell you what not to write!

Hitting the Right Notes in Your Statement

The requirements for your personal statement are precise:

- ✔ **It can't be longer than 47 lines and 4,000 characters.** The character limit includes spaces, hyphens, apostrophes and other symbols.

- ✔ **The line and character limits work independently of each other.** That means that you can't have a statement that's under 4,000 characters but longer than 47 lines, or one that's more than 4,000 characters but under 47 lines.

The space allocated to the personal statement in the UCAS form is formatted so that the 47-line and 4,000-character limits are synchronised. This is probably not the case in the word processing program that you use to draft the statement.

When you finish your draft and paste it into the UCAS form, check that it still meets the line and character limit and that the end hasn't been inadvertently truncated.

Structuring your statement

A good structure to your personal statement allows you to communicate the maximum amount of information to interview shortlisters in the limited space allowed.

You can structure your personal statement in a number of different ways. Although a small number of people advocate a terse bullet-point style, most advise using a narrative format. We definitely support the latter approach and strongly advise against the bullet-point style. The reason is simple: narrative formats – when done well – are more enjoyable to read and easier on the eye. Also, a narrative structure demonstrates your written communication skills, which medical schools value highly.

A narrative structure means telling a coherent story about you and your decision to apply to medical school. It needs to include how you tested your decision and how that proves your suitability to study medicine as a degree and pursue it as a subsequent career.

Break the narrative format down into the following elements and arrange these points into paragraphs as shown:

- ✔ **Introduction (Paragraph 1):** An initial single sentence to engage the reader.

- ✔ **Why medicine (also Paragraph 1):** A summary of the reasons you want to be a doctor.

- ✔ **Commitment to medicine (Paragraph 2):** Your work experience and what you discovered from it that makes you a better candidate.

- ✔ **Non-academic pursuits (Paragraph 3):** Focusing on how they tie into the skills required to be a medical student and doctor.

- ✔ **Personal qualities (also Paragraph 3):** Any talents not already mentioned that support your candidacy.

- ✔ **Gap year (optional; Paragraph 3):** If you're taking a gap year, describe your plans.

- ✔ **Conclusion (Paragraph 4):** A brief summary of your suitability and passion for medicine.

Don't skip the introduction or the conclusion for want of space. These elements give your personal statement a beginning and an end, transforming it into a coherent story. Without them, statements feel like they're 'hanging in mid-air'.

Being precise about the relative lengths of the different paragraphs is difficult because they vary according to what you've actually done. However, as a rough guide allocate as follows:

- ✔ **Paragraph 1:** 20 per cent of your statement

- ✔ **Paragraph 2:** 35 per cent

- ✔ **Paragraph 3:** 35 per cent

- ✔ **Paragraph 4:** 10 per cent

If you're not doing a gap year, reallocate its character count evenly between the other paragraphs.

Knowing what to include

After deciding on the structure of your statement (as we describe in the preceding section), you face the tricky task of fleshing it out with words. A blank page or computer screen is very intimidating and the temptation is to procrastinate until inspiration strikes. This line of thinking goes, 'When I'm in the right mood, the words will just flow and then all I need to do is edit it down a bit'.

This approach never works out well. Good writing is the result of time and discipline; in order to be a writer, you have to write. That means sitting down and forcing yourself to get scribbling. The earlier you start working on your personal statement, the better the eventual product will be.

Prepare for the task as you'd revise for an exam: take it seriously, plan ahead, put in the hours and eventually you'll get a good result.

Take your personal statement as seriously as you do your A-levels. After all, the exam results mean nothing if you don't get shortlisted for an interview.

Presenting your commitment, skills and personal qualities

The following exercise helps you produce material for Paragraphs 2 and 3 of your personal statement:

1. **Carry out the brainstorming (that we describe in Chapter 4) of your different activities and work experience, and how they relate to medical school and being a doctor.** You now have a long list of activities, experiences and personal qualities. If you haven't done that exercise yet, go to Chapter 4 and work through the steps.

2. **Look through the different activities and tease out similar themes.** For example, group together anything that highlights communication skills, leadership qualities or a hard-working and committed ethos.

3. **Rearrange these groupings (on a fresh page) so that they fall under the paragraph headings we mention in the earlier 'Structuring your statement' section.** This method enables you to generate a lot of raw material for Paragraphs 2 and 3, together with a smaller amount for Paragraph 1.

4. **Edit down your raw material.** Eliminate duplication between the paragraphs and focus on particularly rewarding activities that taught you fresh skills or resulted in new insights, especially ones that you can talk about at interview. Aim to highlight activities that demonstrate more than one quality at a time so as to constrain the word count

5. **Start drafting Paragraphs 2 and 3 based on the headings generated by this exercise.**

This method helps you get past any initial writer's block or reluctance to start working on your personal statement. It also forces you to eliminate extraneous material ruthlessly by focusing on the most rewarding activities for each theme. Paragraphs 2 and 3 form the bulk of your statement and so getting started on them first helps you feel that you're making good progress.

Answering why medicine is right for you

After doing the exercise in the preceding section, you still need material for the second half of Paragraph 1 which is about why you want to study medicine. Here are two basic strategies you can employ to answer this question:

- ✔ **The story:** Some people genuinely have an event, or series of events, that they can point to and say that it inspired them to think of medicine as a career. If this applies to you, using this story is a great way to highlight your passion for medicine. Be sure to use the rest of your statement to ground this initial inspiration in a careful exploration of medicine as a career, or else you risk coming across as unrealistic or naïve.

- ✔ **The logical elimination of alternatives:** Not everyone who becomes a good doctor has a dramatic story to tell about why they did so. For many people, the process is quieter and more reflective. They look at their talents and personal qualities and match those traits against a range of professions and find that medicine is the best fit. This is a perfectly acceptable rationale for choosing medicine, but you do need to counterbalance this hard-headed decision making with a zest of passion for medicine elsewhere in your statement.

Both strategies essentially touch upon the same combination of inspiration and commitment to answer the question of why you're applying to study medicine; they just come at the question from opposite angles. The story strategy starts with inspiration, before backing it up with commitment. Logical elimination begins with commitment, before bolstering it with inspiration. This nuanced balance of passion and hard work makes for a good medical student or doctor, and both strategies highlight these traits.

 Incorporate a strand into your explanation that emphasises the importance of communication skills and an interest in working with people.

 The explanation you use in your personal statement should also form the basis of your answer if asked 'Why medicine?' at a later interview. Therefore, ensure that it makes sense to you as an individual. The best explanation is usually the truth, but presented in a way that suit your needs.

Starting and finishing your statement

The introduction and conclusion (Paragraphs 1 and 4) are challenging elements of your statement and we recommend that you think about them last. They need to be brief and engaging, without being 'gimmicky' or overly dramatic. Avoid opening statements rampant with Bulwer-Lytton clichés and purple prose, for example:

It was a dark and stormy night as I lay awake pondering what career to pursue. With a sudden clarity matched only by the flashes of lightning raging outside, I knew that Medicine would be my life's passion. . .

Okay that's an exaggeration of what even the most fevered mind could create as an opening sentence, but the point is that histrionic openings come off as affected and strained. Try instead to come up with a start that's engaging but serious and a conclusion that concisely summarises your intent to study medicine and become a doctor.

Practising Your Writing Skills

Applicants to medical school tend to have strong science backgrounds. As science A-levels require relatively little essay writing compared to the humanities, many candidates are rusty writers. If this applies to you, ensure that it doesn't become apparent in your personal statement. Addressing this potential weakness will give you that extra edge, as a well-written personal statement can really make you stand out from the crowd.

Good writing is a skill that all doctors need. Whether producing patient notes and letters to GPs or drafting research papers and reports for management meetings, the ability to write well is tremendously helpful.

This section can't take the place of writing experience, but we do highlight some principles of good writing that you can apply in your personal statement and in your career.

Writing correctly

Writing correctly means eliminating spelling mistakes, using correct punctuation and minimising grammatical errors. Professional writers have the benefit of copyeditors and proofreaders; we're certainly grateful for all their help with this book! You can access similar help if you get others to check your personal statement before submitting it. Perhaps ask an English teacher at your school to review your personal statement for grammatical and spelling mistakes. If you've left school, maybe ask a friend or two who do a lot of writing in their jobs.

Use full sentences, avoiding abbreviations that the shortlister may not understand. You'd think it obvious not to use slang or 'txt speech', but our experience suggests that it bears saying anyway. Contractions are acceptable because they make the statement feel more immediate, but do use them correctly.

If you use a computerised spellchecker, set it to *English (UK)* not *English (US)*. Double-check suggested corrections because not all spellcheckers are entirely reliable.

We doubt you'll need to use many colons, semi-colons, dashes or parentheses. In fact, we'd go so far as to say you probably won't need any if you follow the advice in this chapter. Instead, break up long sentences into several shorter ones. If you need a quick reminder, Table 5-1 explains the basic functions of some frequently-misused punctuation marks.

Table 5-1	Basic Punctuation Guide
Punctuation Mark	*Function*
Full stop (.)	1.To end a sentence.
	2. To indicate abbreviated words, unless the first and last letters of the word are shown (for example, 'Dr' doesn't require a full stop).
Comma (,)	To separate information (whether lists or phrases) into readable components.
Apostrophe (')	1. In contractions, to indicate missing letters, for example 'can't', 'won't'.
	2. In possessives, to indicate ownership, for example 'Einstein's Theory of Relativity'.
	Note: *its* is possessive but *it's* means *it is* or *it has*.
Colon (:)	1. To indicate the start of a list or summary.
	2. To separate one clause from another, where the second clause supports the first.
Semi-colon (;)	1. To separate what would otherwise stand as individual sentences, but that the author wants to link in meaning.
	2. As a second level of punctuation to separate phrases if commas have already been deployed within the sentence.
Parentheses ( )	To separate out nonessential information in a sentence.
Exclamation mark (!)	To indicate surprise, shock or emphasis.

Producing efficient writing

Efficient writing conveys the maximum amount of information with the fewest words: it's accurate, precise and doesn't waste characters on empty words. When writing against a character limit, efficiency is of paramount importance.

Efficient writing is greatly facilitated by careful structuring, drafting and editing. This preparation allows you to decide what you want to say and the order in which you say it, and gives you the opportunity to rewrite, excising superfluous words and phrases.

 Breaking up long, multi-clausal sentences into several shorter ones is a good way of simplifying your statement and increasing its impact on the reader.

This doesn't mean that efficient writing is fragmented like an old telegram. It features full sentences and good continuity from one paragraph to the next. For example, you might start the paragraph on work experience with something that explains how it follows logically from the preceding paragraph about your decision to study medicine. Even something as simple as, 'Therefore, I decided to find out what a career in medicine involves. . .' introduces this narrative continuity and makes the statement read well.

The final product of your careful editing and rewriting should be a satisfying personal statement that's engaging to read and presents a powerful, concise and logical summary of why you'd be an ideal medical student.

Using active phrasing

The active voice makes your writing more immediate, alive and easier to read. In the active voice, the subject performs the action of the verb, whereas in the passive voice the subject is acted upon. For example:

- ✔ **Active:** 'I saw a patient in my outpatient clinic'.
- ✔ **Passive:** 'A patient was seen by me in my outpatient clinic'.

The active voice makes sentences direct and clear. The passive voice tends to make sentences longer and more opaque. Both forms are grammatically correct, but the active voice is more interesting and immediate to read.

This advice is important in your personal statement because shortlisters read a large number of statements and must quickly decide whether or not to put applicants forward for interview.

More immediate sentences let shortlisters identify key information quicker, boosting your chances of scoring points.

 Students writing personal statements often want to sound 'intelligent'. This can result in overly formal sentences in the passive voice, seasoned with long, pretentious, and often inappropriate words. In fact, short, direct and active sentences come across as much more genuine and convincing.

Selling Yourself to Interview Shortlisters

To whittle down the thousands of applications they receive to a few hundred (at most), medical schools employ a *shortlisting* process. This typically involves several people reading each statement and scoring it against specific criteria, and your task in writing the personal statement is to meet these criteria. This is all about using language and content to present yourself in a truthful but optimal light.

Knowing who reads your statement

Medical schools employ various people to read personal statements, and have differing formulae to score or assess these. In some schools, shortlisters are your potential teachers, such as doctors, professors or fellows. In other institutions, they may be admissions tutors or even administrators with no practical knowledge of medicine.

The good news is that the strategies for structuring a personal statement and writing well (that we describe in the earlier sections 'Hitting the Right Notes in Your Statement' and 'Practising Your Writing Skills', respectively) are valid regardless of who reads your statement. Direct, efficient and structured writing allows anyone to understand the points you're making and grade them quickly against whatever marking scheme they are using.

Using shortlisting to your advantage

Shortlisting culls as many as 80 per cent of applicants, which means that a good personal statement is a powerful tool to boost your chances of getting into medical school. It's an opportunity to shine and demonstrate to medical schools that you have a firm grasp of your own strengths, and how they relate to the attributes that medical schools are looking for.

To give you some examples of how best to make that case, here are some sample excerpts.

An important caveat: *don't copy* these excerpts for your own statement. Not only are they too generic for individual cases, but UCAS uses copy-detection software that flags up any such plagiarism.

Instead, try to understand how we use language to highlight the personal traits that universities are looking for. We place the subtextual message that the text generates in square brackets:

> When my father was taken to hospital with chest pain, I witnessed the incredible work that doctors do, and this inspired me to look into medicine as a career [good solid introduction, setting the scene for the statement and providing a logical inspiration for first looking at medicine as a career]. I was particularly impressed by the doctors' calm and reassuring approach *[awareness of importance of communication skills]*, their skill in taking a history and carrying out a physical examination and their ability to apply their knowledge and powers of deduction to reach the correct diagnosis and treatment plan *[grasp of the basic structure of a medical interview and the scientific model that doctors use].*
>
> *I therefore decided to find out more about what a career in medicine might involve* [linking statement making the narrative flow from the previous paragraph and showing a logical progression of ideas]. *This year I've spent most of my Sunday afternoons at a local hospice* [willingness to give time and effort to others], *working with elderly people with dementia* [unglamorous but important side of medicine]. *Despite the progressive nature of their illness* [demonstrating some medical knowledge], *I found that talking to them, getting them involved in activities and teaching them basic skills can make a significant difference to their quality of life* [good practical experience of medicine, plus an awareness that you can't always cure but you can still make a positive difference]. *These sometimes difficult challenges* [medicine is stressful] *increased my confidence and communication skills* [demonstrating personal insight and talent through anecdote], *and taught me the importance of relying on members of the multidisciplinary team for advice and support* [awareness of teamworking and familiarity with some medical jargon]. *During my summer holidays last year, I spent a month working as a receptionist at a GP practice* [shows you've worked in a range of settings]. *This involved. . .*
>
> *On the social side, I have always been active in extracurricular activities such as the Duke of Edinburgh Award. I'm also a member of my school's chess club and football committees* [demonstrating the ability to work in both solitary and team settings, and the different traits involved]. *I really enjoy these activities because they give me the opportunity to socialise with*

different people and constantly challenge myself to achieve more [communication skills and commitment]. *They also give me a good opportunity to use my creative side and my sense of initiative and innovation* [more demonstration of rounded skills through fact]. *Apart from the above, I cook, sing and play the piano in my spare time, which helps me relax and cope under stress* [importance of relaxation and a healthy work/life balance]. *After my exams I would like to spend the summer travelling. I'm particularly interested in South America and I may be able to organise a long trip to Ecuador where I would be able to combine a holiday with an involvement in charity work* [even on holiday, able to think of others and be generally considerate].

When drafting your own statement, try to use similar techniques to subtextually emphasise your skills, personal progress and general suitability for a career in medicine.

Avoiding Statement Pitfalls

When reviewing personal statements, we see certain repeated errors. Although some of the pitfalls we list may seem trivial or obvious, they do crop up with regular frequency.

Here are some common mistakes that we see all too often:

- ✔ **Focusing excessively on schoolwork:** The UCAS form already includes a separate section listing your educational achievements. Unless you've won a unique or prestigious prize that's not mentioned elsewhere, avoid wasting words on your academic ability.

- ✔ **Concentrating too much on future career plans:** At your stage, you're unlikely to have enough practical experience to make definitive statements about future career plans, especially if they're in a super-specialised field. If you like the idea of becoming a GP by all means suggest that you're looking forward to that rotation, but much more than that can come across as naive and presumptuous.

- ✔ **Giving yourself the hard sell:** Avoid non-evidenced statements such as 'I have excellent communication skills'. Instead, demonstrate your communication skills by giving concrete examples of times when you demonstrated those skills. Flip to the earlier section 'Selling Yourself to Interview Shortlisters' for more advice on this topic.

- ✔ **Using the royal we:** The personal statement is yours and so you're allowed to write 'I' rather than 'we'. Too much use of 'we' comes across as lacking in confidence. As in the preceding point, however, the best statements always support declarations of personal achievement or ability with evidence.

✔ **Providing silly reasons for studying medicine:** These include, but aren't limited to, inanities such as 'it's a respectable career', 'it's a secure job with a good salary', 'my mother/father/brother is a doctor so I know what the job entails', 'I got straight As and A*s in my GCSEs and A-level predictions' and 'I don't want to be a lawyer or accountant'. The first two answers are too self-serving, the third comes across as nepotistic and the last two aren't positive choices in favour of being a doctor.

If you come from a medical family and want to leverage the experience you gained as a result, talk about all the wonderful things you discovered during your work experience. Just don't mention how you came to get that experience!

The 'I don't want to be a lawyer or accountant' response differs from the logical elimination strategy we describe earlier in the chapter in 'Answering why medicine is for you'. Logical elimination is a positive choice demonstrating good personal insight; you took a good hard look at yourself and decided medicine would make the best use of your talents. The 'don't want to be a lawyer or accountant' statement is only negative.

✔ **Being boring:** To avoid this fate, read the earlier sections 'Practising Your Writing Skills' and 'Selling Yourself to Interview Shortlisters'.

✔ **Bad writing:** Poor grammar and punctuation confuses and distracts shortlisters. They may have thousands of statements to read and if they can't get the facts from your statement quickly, they're likely to assume that none exist and score you down. Check out 'Practising Your Writing Skills' earlier in this chapter to bone up on good-writing techniques.

✔ **Copying:** UCAS uses advanced anti-plagiarism software to detect copying of other people's statements, from the current cycle or previous years. This software also cross-references your statement against common sources, such as the Internet. In short, don't copy. In any event, copied statements can never be specific to your own skills and experiences, and so you're actually doing yourself a disservice.

✔ **Lying:** This is the worst thing you can do in a personal statement. Not only do you get caught out if you're asked about the topic in an interview, but also doctors – and by extension, you – are supposed to be honest people. Lives can depend on it.

Part II
Sitting the Tests

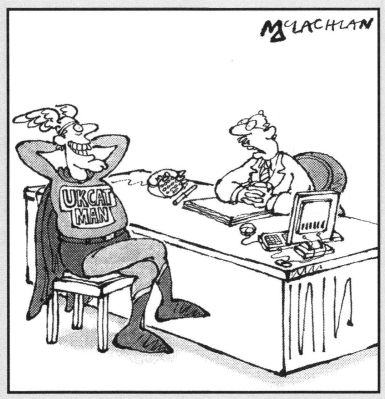

"Pretty confident, aren't you, Mr. Tollboothe."

In this part...

Part II focuses on the three selection tests that UK medical schools ask candidates to sit.

Each test is reviewed in turn, starting with the UKCAT, moving onto the BMAT and ending with the GAMSAT. For the two most common selection tests, the UKCAT and BMAT, we also provide a small selection of practice questions to give you a flavour of the challenges that lie ahead, together with full answers and explanations.

Study this part carefully to get a head start on your competition.

Chapter 6

Dissecting the UKCAT

. . . .

In This Chapter

▶ Introducing the UKCAT

▶ Sitting and applying for the test

▶ Revealing the test's structure

▶ Getting to know the subtests

. . . .

*M*any medical schools (which we identify in this chapter) require applicants to sit the United Kingdom Clinical Aptitude Test (UKCAT) as part of their selection procedures. Most students find that the five subtests of the UKCAT form a challenging and novel test.

To help with your preparation and revision, we discuss the nature of the UKCAT, the application process and its overall structure. We also describe the various subtests in detail and provide tips to increase your chances of a successful outcome.

Exploring the UKCAT

The UKCAT is a test of aptitude and is theoretically designed to reward candidates with a natural talent for the tested skills.

The universities that request it already have lots of information about applicants' current academic achievements in the form of GCSE and A-level (or Scottish Higher) results and predictions, but wish to assess a wider range of intellectual abilities identified as being useful in medicine, including critical thinking, logical reasoning and inference.

These universities hope that an aptitude test – the results of which they consider alongside the pre-existing academic record – can help them choose the most suitable candidates to join their medical and dental courses. They also hope that the UKCAT is a fairer way of narrowing down the applicant field. Aptitude tests are relatively good predictors of underlying talent and minimise the effects of background and schooling on a candidate's academic achievement. For more information about the potential validity of the UKCAT, see the sidebar 'Does the UKCAT work?'.

The UKCAT is a *psychometric test*. It tries to measure your thought processes or, more accurately, how those thought processes affect your performance on a set of standardised tasks. By grouping those tasks into different subtests, the results show the examiner how your ability varies across different dimensions of intellectual ability.

Considering the UKCAT Process

The UKCAT is designed for applicants to medical and dental university courses. The test is a required part of the selection process for the courses and universities listed in Table 6-1. Table 6-2 expands on the UCAS (Universities and Colleges Admissions Service) course codes in Table 6-1.

Table 6-1	Universities and Courses that Require the UKCAT
University	**UCAS Course Code**
Aberdeen	A100, A201
Brighton and Sussex Medical School	A100
Barts and The London School of Medicine and Dentistry	A100, A101, A200, A201
Cardiff	A100, A104, A200, A204
Dundee	A100, A104, A200, A204
Durham	A100
East Anglia	A100, A104
Edinburgh	A100
Glasgow	A100, A200
Hull York Medical School	A100
Keele	A100, A104
King's College London	A100, A101, A102, A202, A205

University	UCAS Course Code
Imperial College London Graduate Entry	A101
Leeds	A100
Leicester	A100, A101
Manchester	A104, A106, A204, A206
Newcastle	A100, A101, A206
Nottingham	A100, A108
Peninsula College of Medicine and Dentistry	A100
Queen's University Belfast	A100, A200
Sheffield	A100, A104, A200
Southampton	A100, A101, A102
St Andrews	A100, A990, B900
St George's, University of London	A100
Warwick University Graduate Entry	A101

Table 6-2   UCAS Course Codes

UCAS Code	Course
A100	Medicine
A101	Medicine (graduate entry 4-year programmes everywhere, except King's Extended Medical Degree)
A102	Medicine (widening access 6-year programme at Southampton; graduate professional entry 4-year programme at King's)
A104	Medicine (including initial pre-medical/foundation year)
A108	Medicine (including foundation year, Nottingham only)
A200	Dentistry
A201	Dentistry (graduate entry 4-year programmes)

(continued)

Table 6-2 *(continued)*

UCAS Code	Course
A204	Dentistry (including pre-dental/foundation year, except King's, where it's for medical graduates)
A205	Dentistry (King's only)
A206	Dentistry (Newcastle and Manchester)
A990	North American Medical Programme (St Andrews only)
B900	International Foundation for Medicine (St Andrews only, 1-year programme)

In short, the UKCAT is required for undergraduate medical entry everywhere in the UK except Cambridge, Imperial, Oxford and University College London (which require the BMAT, described in Chapter 8) and Birmingham, Bristol, Liverpool and Swansea. Note that Imperial and Warwick do require the UKCAT for their graduate medical courses.

Finding out whether you're exempt from taking the UKCAT

You have to sit the UKCAT if your chosen institution and course are listed in Tables 6-1 and 6-2, and you live and are educated in one of the following countries:

Australia, Austria, Bahrain, Bangladesh, Belgium, Botswana, Brunei, Bulgaria, Cameroon, Canada, China, Cyprus, Czech Republic, Denmark, Egypt, Estonia, Finland, France, Germany, Ghana, Gibraltar, Greece, Hong Kong, Hungary, India, Indonesia, Ireland, Israel, Italy, Japan, Jordan, Kenya, Kuwait, Latvia, Lithuania, Luxembourg, Malaysia, Malta, Mauritius, Netherlands, New Zealand, Nigeria, Norway, Pakistan, Poland, Portugal, Qatar, Republic of Korea, Romania, Saudi Arabia, Singapore, Slovakia, Slovenia, South Africa, Spain, Sri Lanka, Sweden, Switzerland, Taiwan, Thailand, Uganda, United Arab Emirates, United Kingdom of Great Britain and Northern Ireland, United Republic of Tanzania and the United States of America.

If your home isn't in one of the countries listed above, you're exempt from sitting the UKCAT. You still need to fill in a form, however, that you can easily find on the UKCAT website (www.ukcat.ac.uk). You are then issued with a reference number and your chosen universities are informed of your exemption.

Does the UKCAT work?

Debate surrounds whether the UKCAT succeeds in its aim of testing underlying aptitude and whether its inclusion in the selection process adds to its fairness.

In its favour, the test doesn't contain any curriculum or science content. It focuses on the cognitive areas it aims to test. The UKCAT Consortium takes great care to ensure that the test questions are written by appropriate experts. It then tests the questions extensively for validity and reliability and attempts to minimise cultural bias.

Critics point out that the very existence of the UKCAT introduces an extra hurdle. People from backgrounds not historically likely to apply to medical schools may be put off by having to sit yet another exam, whereas people from schools or families with experience of the system may be more confident of gaming it. In addition, the UKCAT has an entrance fee of £65 or £80 (or £100 for non-EU candidates), depending on when you sit the exam, which may prevent some people from registering to take it. Bursaries to cover the cost are available in some circumstances, and we provide more details on this aspect and the fees in the later section 'Uncovering the UKCAT registration process'.

More fundamentally, critics question how valid an aptitude test the UKCAT really is. If it were purely testing aptitude, then you would score the same regardless of whether and how much you had prepared. The UKCAT Consortium takes great pains to emphasise that you don't need to prepare for the test and yet its own website states: 'You should take the time to familiarise yourself with the test. We strongly advise you to practise answering the types of questions that will be presented in the UKCAT, to familiarise yourself with the question styles, multiple-choice format and varying requirements of each subtest.' Re-applicant candidates tend to improve their scores in the second year, which again implies that familiarity and practice improves performance. The bottom line is that revising for the UKCAT significantly improves your chances of getting into medical school.

Noting the crucial dates

You have to take the UKCAT in the year of your application cycle. For example, candidates applying in 2013 for entry in 2014 (or for deferred entry in 2015) must sit the UKCAT in 2013. Your test score is valid only for one application cycle. If you reapply the following year, you need to sit the UKCAT all over again.

The logic behind the need to re-sit an aptitude test from one year to the next somewhat escapes us: aptitude is innate and shouldn't vary significantly from one year to the next. Nonetheless, the UKCAT rules are very clear about re-sitting, and so be sure to stick to them.

The exact dates for the UKCAT registration, testing and publication-of-results cycle vary from year to year, though usually only by a day or two. The organisers maintain a good website with the relevant dates for the current year (www.ukcat.ac.uk) and loads of other useful information as well.

As a general guide, Table 6-3 shows the important dates for a typical cycle.

Table 6-3	The UKCAT Dates for a Typical Cycle
Event	*Date*
Registration opens	1 May
Bursary applications open	1 May
Testing begins	3 July
Registration deadline	21 September
Bursary application deadline	21 September
Exemption application deadline	21 September
Last testing date	5 October
UCAS application deadline	15 October

 We recommend that you aim to sit the UKCAT fairly early in the cycle. Then, if you fall ill or for some other reason can't make your initial test date, you still have time to rebook to a later date. This approach also puts the UKCAT test date a safe distance from that for the BMAT (discussed in Chapter 8). That way, if you have to sit both tests you have the time and mental space to prepare thoroughly for each.

An early test date does mean that you have to start your preparation sooner, but the insurance you gain by having room to manoeuvre is probably worth the trade-off.

 If you need to cancel or reschedule your test, log into Pearson VUE's website (www.pearsonvue.co.uk). Rescheduling is free of charge, provided this is done a full working day prior to the original test date. Otherwise you're counted as a no-show and are liable for the full fee – and then have to pay a further fee for the rescheduled test.

Uncovering the UKCAT registration process

UKCAT registration is entirely computerised. Go to UKCAT's website at www.ukcat.ac.uk and click Sign In at the top of the page or the Register Here link under Quick Links. Registration is possible only within the period indicated in Table 6-3. You're seamlessly transferred to Pearson VUE's website and guided through a series of online forms to create an account to access the system, register and pay for the test. Registering is no more intimidating than opening an account with any online shopping site, so don't panic!

The application fee is £65 if you sit the test in the summer and £80 if you sit it in the autumn. If you're not from an EU country, the fee rises to £100, regardless of when you sit the test. Payment is made online with any major credit or debit card. There is, unfortunately, no other way: if you don't have access to a credit or debit card, look into getting a temporary or prepaid card from your bank or from other organisations such as the Post Office.

Many potentially eligible applicants don't realise that an extensive bursary system operates that covers many EU candidates for the full cost of the test fee. In fact, poor level of awareness around the bursary system was one of the areas highlighted in a candidate survey carried out by UKCAT. You can apply for a bursary by completing the form at www.ukcat.ac.uk/registration/bursaries/bursary-application-form. You can only apply during the registration window indicated in Table 6-3.

Historically, bursaries were available for those in receipt of the Educational Maintenance Allowance (EMA) or Adult Learning Grant (ALG). Recipients of Income Support, 16–19 Bursary Fund and some other benefits were also eligible for bursaries. EMA and ALG are now closed, and at the time of writing, UKCAT hasn't confirmed the new requirements that are going to govern future bursary awards. Check the bursary website when the application period opens for the very latest information.

The process of applying for a bursary requires documentary evidence (generally a letter from the relevant government agency) to verify your eligibility. Once you demonstrate eligibility, UKCAT sends you a voucher code that you can then enter into the online booking system. The processes for future bursaries are likely to be similar, with only the details of the eligible benefits changing.

If you've already paid, you may still be able to get a refund. Contact Pearson VUE Customer Services directly on +44 (0) 161 855 7409.

If you're able to demonstrate that you have special educational needs such as dyslexia, dysgraphia, or attention deficit hyperactivity disorder, you can sit the UKCATSEN in lieu of the UKCAT. The UKCATSEN is exactly the same as the UKCAT but with 25 per cent more time to complete the exam. Mobility and other needs are also catered for as long as prior notice is received.

Don't register for the UKCATSEN if you don't have special educational needs. Not only would such behavior be unethical, but you would get caught out. Although UKCAT doesn't expect you to provide clinical evidence to verify your eligibility for UKCATSEN, the universities do. Your test results are declared null and void if you're unable to provide this evidence. The evidence needed is typically in the form of a certificate from a qualified medical practitioner or other relevant health professional.

Tackling the UKCAT on the day

You can find UKCAT centres across the UK and in the countries where UKCAT isn't exempted (see the earlier section 'Finding out whether you're exempt from taking the UKCAT'). You should be able to find one relatively close to you via the UKCAT website (www.ukcat.ac.uk).

Check out where you need to go on test day! We can't think of anything worse than turning up to an exam late, or rushing to get there and then feeling frazzled, sweaty and confused. For the UKCAT, we recommend being 15–30 minutes early, because you need to go through some formalities before you start the exam.

Bring photographic proof of identity with you, such as a valid adult passport with your own signature (children's passports aren't accepted) or a photocard driving licence. If you have neither of these documents, ask your school to provide an appropriately certified form letter.

You don't need to take anything else with you. In fact, you're not permitted to take anything else into the test room itself. This prohibition includes coats, bags, phones, wallets, watches, keys and sweets. This may seem rather draconian, but at least you've been forewarned – don't wear your priceless family heirloom Rolex because the invigilator will insist you leave it in a locker.

For the exam your workstation consists of a computer, a laminated non-erasable notepad and pen, and a chair. You can ask for a set of headphones or earplugs if the ambient noise is too loud. UKCAT recently revised its procedures to avoid the need to issue handheld calculators to candidates. Instead, you now have access to a software-based calculator on your workstation computer (for more details, check out the later section 'Finding out the format of the Quantitative Reasoning subtest').

You can leave the room for invigilator-escorted comfort breaks, but the test isn't paused during this time. So make sure to go to the loo before the exam. The time pressure is already one of the toughest things about the exam and you don't want to make it worse. As the UKCAT is computer-marked, you will receive your results immediately after having sat the test.

The UKCAT organisers automatically forward the results to the relevant universities on your UKCAT form. If you want an extra transcript of your results, you can order one for a fee of £25.

You can't retake the test in the same application cycle.

Unveiling the UKCAT's Overall Structure

The UKCAT is a computer-administered exam lasting two hours. The test consists of five parts or subtests: Verbal Reasoning, Quantitative Reasoning, Abstract Reasoning, Decision Analysis and Situational Judgement. Each of the five subtests is in a multiple-choice format and is timed separately. This section covers the timings and scoring of the UKCAT. (For details of the five subtests, flip to the later section 'Examining the Subtests'.)

Thinking about the timing

Students consistently report that one of the hardest things about the UKCAT is the time pressure and not the content. So that you know what's expected of you, Table 6-4 shows the timings for the UKCAT and the number of question items in each section.

The times per item give you a general idea of how to pace yourself through each subtest, though remember that you may need to spend a little more time on the harder questions and as little as possible on the simpler ones. The UKCAT is designed to allow the very best candidates to complete the entire test, although the pace required to do so is challenging.

If you sit the UKCATSEN (which we describe earlier in the 'Uncovering the UKCAT registration process' section), you do have an extra 25 per cent of time for each section. The UKCATSEN is otherwise identical to the UKCAT.

Table 6-4	Timings for the UKCAT Subtests		
Subtest	*Time Allowed*	*Number of Items*	*Time per Item*
Verbal Reasoning	22 minutes	44 items	30 seconds
Quantitative Reasoning	23 minutes	36 items	38 seconds
Abstract Reasoning	16 minutes	65 items	15 seconds
Decision Analysis	32 minutes	26 items	74 seconds
Situational Judgement	27 minutes	60 items	27 seconds

 You're one step ahead if you realise that practising any test, even the UKCAT, results in better test scores. Familiarising yourself with the pace required is an essential component of your revision. Our *UKCAT For Dummies* (Wiley) book contains multiple complete timed practice tests to help you with your revision. The practice tests at www.ukcat.ac.uk/preparation/practice-test usefully simulate UKCAT's own computer software, enabling you to familiarise yourself with the practicalities of sitting the exam.

Understanding the marking systems

The UKCAT is marked based on the number of correct responses you give on the test. The test doesn't use *negative marking* and so your score doesn't drop if you give a wrong answer; you just fail to gain a mark on that particular question.

 Guess if you don't know an answer, because you have nothing to lose.

The number of correct responses is scaled into a mark for each of the first four subtests, ranging from 300 to 900. The total score for the entire test therefore ranges from 1200 to 3600. The new Situational Judgement subtest doesn't form part of the selection process in 2012; at time of writing no decision has been taken as to whether (or how) it will contribute to candidates' marks in the future.

The UKCAT doesn't have a specific pass mark, and different universities have different opinions on what they consider to be a good score. (See the following 'Weighing up the scores' section for more on scoring.)

Weighing up the scores

Each university within the UKCAT Consortium is free to decide for itself the importance of your UKCAT score. As a result, significant variation exists in how the various universities weigh your score during their selection processes.

Some universities give the score fairly short shrift, others look at it in conjuction with other criteria and a few consider it to be absolutely vital.

Historically, these UKCAT-heavy universities are Barts and The London, Durham, Glasgow, Hull/York, Queen's University Belfast, Sheffield and Warwick. However, there is a general trend away from using the UKCAT score as a crude cut-off for shortlisting. For example, in 2011 the University of Sheffield used a cut-off total score for shortlisting of 2870, but for 2012 they decided to drop the strict cut-off and use the UKCAT score more flexibly.

Candidates often agonise about this variation between universities, both before and after sitting the test. This is a terrible waste of nervous energy; just do your best, regardless of the precise weighting formula of your preferred university.

Focus on practising as much as you can before the test, staying calm and pacing yourself during the exam. Then put the results out of your mind. After the test, concentrate on the things that are still within your power to improve your odds of getting into medical school, in particular preparing for the interviews (read the chapters in Part III) and keeping up to date with major advances in the world of medicine (Chapter 13).

 Think of the application process as the London Marathon and the UKCAT as the equivalent of crossing Tower Bridge. The UKCAT is an important milestone, but it isn't the end of the race. You can still recover, or indeed fall back, after you sit the UKCAT. After you cross the bridge, put it out of your mind and focus on the rest of the race.

Examining the Subtests

Understanding the structure of the UKCAT is important (as we discuss in the earlier section 'Unveiling the UKCAT's Overall Structure'), but you also need to be familiar with the individual subtests. In this section we go through each subtest in detail.

Turn to Chapter 7 for a selection of sample questions for the Verbal Reasoning, Quantitative Reasoning, Abstract Reasoning and Decision Analysis subtests (we don't supply any for the new Situational Judgement subtest because it's currently under pilot. It may undergo extensive changes before it becomes an official part of the process, rendering any potential sample questions invalid and even misleading). If you want an even larger sample of UKCAT questions, our companion book *UKCAT For Dummies* (Wiley) contains enough practice questions to fill three UKCAT exams, together with answers and explanations.

Getting the message: Verbal Reasoning subtest

Verbal reasoning is the skill with which you understand and work out the meanings of written words, and draw conclusions based on what you read. In short, verbal reasoning is what helps you understand meaning when presented with written or spoken information. You already do this; you've been working on it all your life.

The UKCAT tests your verbal reasoning ability because this skill is vital for any clinician. For example, the average day of a GP starts off slowly with a coffee before catching up on received emails. One message is from a nursing colleague requesting advice about a patient; another is from a manager giving feedback from a recent administrative meeting; and the third contains a pharmacy bulletin about a newly discovered adverse drug reaction.

Verbal reasoning lets the GP quickly read all three messages, determine what each person wants and needs, and work out whether he needs to do anything to keep everyone happy. For instance, he may ask a few pertinent questions to get more details before giving the nurse some advice. He may send the manager a quick confirmation that he's read the email and mention a couple of problems that the administrators need to consider. And the information about the adverse drug reaction may prompt the GP to check that none of his patients on that drug show any early signs of the reaction. Even before seeing his first patient of the day, he's actively used verbal reasoning in his clinical practice.

The UKCAT Verbal Reasoning subtest examines how well you may perform when faced with similar situations in the future. Universities want to see that you can rapidly take on board written information and use it correctly.

Fathoming the format of the Verbal Reasoning subtest

The Verbal Reasoning subtest consists of 11 passages of prose. After each passage come 4 statements referring to the passage – giving a total of 44 statements. You have 22 minutes to complete the subtest.

You have to read each passage, think carefully about the information presented and use the information to answer each statement. You have to determine whether each statement is true or false, or whether you can't tell.

'Can't tell' means that it's impossible to decide on the basis of the information given in the statement whether it's true or false – not that you find the question too difficult to answer.

The Verbal Reasoning subtest examines whether you're able to understand the information provided and logically infer assumptions and conclusions *from that information,* not whether you already know the answers based on your general knowledge. The subtest is about *logic.* This subtle difference is one potential reason why many intelligent and well-read candidates do worse than they expected.

Base your answer solely on the information in the passage. Even if you already know something about the topic discussed in the passage, try to forget that extraneous knowledge and answer each statement using only the information provided. For example, if the text states that London is the capital of France, you need to accept this as fact for the purposes of answering the questions.

Preparing for the Verbal Reasoning subtest

A good way to prepare for the Verbal Reasoning subtest is to practise reading dense, complicated material. Any well-written source of information is fine; the material doesn't have to be about medical matters. In fact, at this early stage in your life, we recommend you try to read as widely as possible as it helps to better understand the world around you.

A great starting point is the broadsheet newspapers: in other words, papers that don't have large supplements on TV talent contests or celebrities. Especially useful are their opinion columns. Broadsheet columnists are paid considerable sums of money to write about topical events and draw parallels and conclusions about them. Most opinion columns are rather biased (because strong opinions help to sell papers), which means that the writers do their best to present a persuasive and logical argument rather than neutral facts. This structure makes them ideal to analyse in the same way as you would a Verbal Reasoning passage.

Read an article and then summarise the information. Keep shrinking down your summary until you remove all irrelevant fluff and meaningless words tugging at the heart or the purse strings (depending on the columnist's political persuasion). Half the time, you uncover conflicting conclusions, which says more about the confused thinking of some columnists than your verbal reasoning ability.

You need to be able to summarise information quickly, stripping the verbose flesh away from the logical bones of a fat passage of purple prose. If you have this ability, you may well find the UKCAT Verbal Reasoning subtest surprisingly simple.

The ability to extract information rapidly from a wide range of sources helps you formulate opinions for yourself, and think widely about the world and its problems. This is a useful trait for any person to have and gives you an unusually lucid and perceptive outlook on life.

Working efficiently on test day

Test day can be unnerving. You can easily lose concentration and start to panic, especially given the intense time pressure of the exam.

The following tips for the Verbal Reasoning subtest help to keep you focused, improve your accuracy and reduce your chances of spending too long on any one question:

- ✔ **Read the passage quickly but carefully.**

- ✔ **Avoid skipping sentences or guessing how they finish.**

- ✔ **Remember that each paragraph of a well-composed passage tends to make one individual, central point.** Try to distill the essential meaning of each paragraph to help you simplify the text in your mind.

- ✔ **Don't skim read because it can force unwarranted assumptions.** When skimming, you unconsciously draw on your background knowledge to fill in the gaps and tend to ignore what's actually written down.

- ✔ **Don't get hung up on things that you know are wrong.** The text isn't designed to be factually correct but to test your ability to reason on the basis of the information provided.

- ✔ **Don't get angry or irritated with an opinion expressed in the passage.** Put your own opinions to one side, stay cool and focus on getting the questions right.

To build up your confidence, practise the sample Verbal Reasoning questions in Chapter 7.

Working with numbers: Quantitative Reasoning subtest

The Quantitative Reasoning subtest assesses how you work with numerical information, and uses examples relevant to the problems doctors have to solve. As someone planning to apply to medical or dental school, you almost certainly already have a good GCSE in maths. The Quantitative Reasoning subtest in the UKCAT doesn't draw on any skills beyond GCSE maths, and so with a little bit of practice you should do really well in this test.

At first glance you may think that the ability to manipulate numbers comfortably has little to do with medicine or dentistry, but maths crops up in all sorts of clinical nooks and crannies. Consider the following example that shows maths at work and saving lives. A doctor is on his ward round, seeing patients. A junior doctor updates him on a particularly unwell patient with a serious infection, reeling off a string of blood test results. The doctor immediately realises that the test results are outside the normal range, and, moreover, that they are considerably worse than the day before. These deductions are basic mathematical operations.

As a result, the doctor decides to switch the patient's antibiotic from an oral tablet to an intravenous infusion, knowing that this is going to be more effective. But the antibiotic is toxic at higher doses. He double-checks the required dose in his formulary and finds that he should base the dose on the patient's weight. He looks this up on the patient's weight chart, uses it to calculate the required total dose and then prescribes it onto the patient's drug chart.

Finding out the format of the Quantitative Reasoning subtest

The UKCAT Quantitative Reasoning subtest consists of nine numerical presentations. After each presentation are 4 questions on the content of the presentation, yielding a total of 36 questions. The test data is presented in the form of tables, charts and graphs and you have to be able to rapidly identify relevant information and then manipulate that information to find the correct answers. You have 23 minutes to complete the subtest.

The testers are looking for basic mathematical capabilities. They want to see that you can:

 ✔ Perform simple mathematical operations

 ✔ Understand proportions, percentages and ratios

 ✔ Apply different kinds of average

✔ Work comfortably with fractions and decimals

✔ Convert from one unit to another

✔ Apply and solve basic equations

The Quantitative Reasoning subtest places more emphasis on using numbers to solve real life problems than on raw mathematical ability. The subtest is checking that you can determine what numbers can reveal (and hide!) as opposed to whether you can number-crunch like a computer.

Most people find that, compared with the other sections of the UKCAT, this subtest is intellectually simpler but harder to complete within the time limit. The key is to remain focused throughout and avoid making silly mathematical errors.

The UKCAT now prohibits the use of handheld calculators and instead provides you with an on-screen calculator with basic functionality. You can access this calculator with the click of an icon and let it run in the background as you move from one question to the next.

Many people find on-screen calculators harder to use than more familiar handheld devices, so do practise using the calculator on your PC. Then do the practice tests on the UKCAT website to familiarise yourself with the real thing (www.ukcat.ac.uk/preparation/practice-test).

Aiming for success in the Quantitative Reasoning subtest

To do well in this subtest, you need to be familiar with certain basic mathematical operations that you may already know from GCSE level mathematics:

✔ Addition, subtraction, multiplication and division

✔ Percentages, ratios and fractions

✔ Speed, distance and time calculations

✔ Working with money

✔ Areas and volumes

✔ Graphs and charts

If you feel rusty working with these simple operations, have a look through your GCSE maths books again and then get up to speed by doing lots of practice questions.

Working well on test day

Follow these simple tips to keep yourself focused, reduce your error rate, and avoid spending too much time on any given question:

- ✔ **Don't be intimidated by presentations on topics you know nothing about.** The testers are looking at how well you can manipulate numerical information, not whether you're familiar with the topic of the presentation.

- ✔ **Practise using the on-screen calculator before test day.** Also, beware of typos while using it. On the day itself, leave yourself some time to double-check the more involved calculations.

- ✔ **Don't overcomplicate the questions.** They require the use of fairly basic mathematical operations. If you have to draw on advanced mathematics in your attempts to solve the problem, you're almost certainly barking up the wrong tree.

- ✔ **Don't be overconfident just because you're already very comfortable working with maths.** Read each question carefully and work steadily to avoid making careless errors. You can easily misinterpret or overlook a vital aspect of the question.

- ✔ **Don't relax too much.** This can lead to careless errors in a subtest on which you would otherwise have scored very highly.

- ✔ **Don't spend too much time on a question you can't solve.** Move on to the next question and keep your cool. You aren't expected to get 100%, so best accept that and use your time to your best advantage.

Practising the sample selection of questions in Chapter 7 might reveal just how easily silly mistakes can be made. Please don't let it be you!

Recognising patterns: Abstract Reasoning subtest

In the Abstract Reasoning subtest you look at two groups of strange-looking diagrams and identify a common pattern (or common patterns) within each group. You are then given five items that you need to fit into one of the groups; some of the items might not fit into either group, in which case the answer is 'can't tell'.

The subtest assesses how you infer relationships from the patterns of abstract shapes. The patterns may include irrelevant and distracting material that has been included as a red herring and that can easily mislead or confuse you.

Many students find the Abstract Reasoning subtest the most intimidating subtest. Whereas other subtests deal with familiar concepts, the abstract reasoning subtest is . . . well . . . abstract. So why has this test been included in an exam for future doctors?

A consultant welcomes a patient into his outpatient clinic. As the patient tells his story, the consultant listens and thinks. He begins to formulate hypotheses about what may be wrong with the patient and decides what questions he needs to ask to either prove or disprove each hypothesis. This makes the consultant very efficient, as he only needs to ask a few precisely targeted questions.

The consultant's way of working feels instinctive to him, but it's actually the product of years of training and experience. The knowledge database that he gradually acquired enables him to recognise patterns, that is, to identify thematic similarities between his patient and countless other patients he's already seen. These similarities help him to form an idea of what the patient might be suffering from, even before carrying out a full history and physical examination. As the patient divulges more information, the consultant uses this data to confirm or reject the various diagnostic possibilities that he initially came up with.

Training and experience has helped the consultant to do this, but the job's easier if he's naturally gifted at this sort of thing. And this is exactly what the Abstract Reasoning subtest measures.

To be successful in this subtest, you have to demonstrate a scientific approach to recognising patterns. You need to create hypotheses quickly and test them against the available information to arrive at the correct answers.

Figuring out the format of the Abstract Reasoning subtest

In this subtest, you are given two sets of shapes, labelled Set A and Set B. The shapes in Set A all have something in common as do the six shapes in Set B. The two sets of shapes aren't related to each other in any way. For each pair of sets, you then see five test shapes. Your task is to decide whether each test shape belongs to Set A, Set B or Neither Set.

The subtest contains 13 set pairs, with 5 test items per pair, for a total of 65 questions. You have just 16 minutes to complete the subtest.

To answer 65 questions in 16 minutes, you need to work at a very fast rate of 4 questions a minute.

Working out patterns in the Abstract Reasoning subtest

You rarely notice the pattern similarity within each set instantly. To speed yourself up, we suggest that you use a common approach to identifying the pattern similarity within each set. With added practice, you might discover your optimal approach to this subtest, but for now work through our list of ideas to focus quickly on the commonality within each set. Applying this list of possible similarities to each set allows you quickly to generate potential hypotheses about the set. You can then test each hypothesis in turn, accepting or discarding hypotheses as applicable. Here's our list of identifiers to look for:

- Shape of components

- Number of sides or corners to each component

- Type of lines or edges on each component, e.g. solid versus dashed, straight versus curved

- Types of angles on each component, e.g. presence of right angles

- Colour of each component, e.g. whether a component is always black or white

- Number of components

- Orientation of components

- Consistent (or consistently evolving) position of one component relative to the others

- Size of components

This list isn't exhaustive, and sometimes more than one rule applies, making the question more complicated. But our suggestions are a good starting point and may get you out of trouble if you're stuck on a question.

Pattern recognition is a function of experience. The more Abstract Reasoning questions you practise, the better you get at doing them.

Coping with the Abstract Reasoning subtest on test day

The Abstract Reasoning subtest is intimidating, and many candidates panic and give up too easily. But this is no wonder given the intense time pressure. The following tips can help you keep your cool:

✔ **Don't be intimidated by a set you can't instantly solve.**
Consider the list of basic commonalities that we mention in
the preceding section and work your way through each possibility. If none of the possibilities fits the set of shapes, move
on to the next question. You can always come back to a
set later on. By moving on, you're maximising your scoring
opportunities.

✔ **Remember that you have more time than you think.** The real
challenge of the subtest is in identifying the commonalities,
not in answering the actual questions. So think in terms of
time per set rather than time per question. After you spot the
commonality in a set, working through each test shape and
seeing which set it belongs to is usually quick and easy.

✔ **Accept that some of the sets are very complex.** The sets
toward the end of the subtest are particularly complicated,
with multiple interacting features. Few people solve these
questions correctly, and so don't be surprised or worried if
you can't manage them.

✔ **Be wary of red herrings.** Look out for features that appear to
present an answer but that don't quite work out. Check your
rule: if it is 100% correct, then there should be no exceptions
at all.

✔ **Take a few deep breaths and mentally set the test aside if
you feel you've done badly in it.** The UKCAT tests a range of
different aptitudes and very few people excel at all of them.
Shift your attention to the subtest and do your very best
on that.

The sample questions and answers in Chapter 7 enable you to
experience how quick and easy it is to answer the questions once
you have uncovered the commonality.

Making up your mind: Decision Analysis subtest

Diagnosing patients and allocating valuable medical resources
requires quick decision-making skills. The Decision Analysis subtest checks whether you have the innate aptitude to make such
decisions.

This subtest is all about making judgement calls. You have to use a
code to unscramble coded phrases into English and, conversely, to
encode English phrases into the code. At first glance, the concept
is straightforward. The catch is that the code lacks the breadth
you need to translate fully and explicitly to and from English. The
code covers concepts rather than letters, and for that reason

translation is as much an exercise in manipulating concepts as in looking up items in the code. Playing around with concepts and manipulating their meaning requires good judgement, which is exactly what the subtest is examining.

Here's an example of how decision analysis is relevant to the work of a doctor. A consultant is on duty one evening, answering GPs who are calling to refer patients, that is, to ask the hospital duty team to see certain patients.

A GP calls to say that he has a patient in his surgery with leg weakness. He's concerned that the patient may be having a stroke and would like to send him to hospital for further tests and treatment. Though the GP has taken a thorough history and examined the patient, he lacks the diagnostic and therapeutic facilities that are available at the hospital. The consultant and the GP discuss the patient over the phone. The GP doesn't have all the data to know for sure whether the patient needs hospital treatment. The patient may have had a stroke – but he may also have a less urgent complaint.

The consultant triages (grades) the urgency of the patient's symptoms on the basis of the limited information provided by the GP, slotting that information into the conceptual framework that he has learnt through years of training and experience. Not to see a patient with a serious, life-threatening condition no doubt constitutes negligence, but seeing patients with non-urgent complaints takes time away from more seriously ill people.

Decoding the format of the Decision Analysis subtest

In this subtest, you have to read a scenario and then answer 26 questions based on the scenario. You have 32 minutes to complete the subtest. The scenario typically involves a brief paragraph of prose outlining the basic context of the scenario, followed by a table full of data. The questions concern codes constructed from the data in the table.

Unlike with other subtests, more than one of four or five response options may be correct. The question will state whether you need to select more than one answer, in which case one mark is awarded for getting both answers right and no marks are awarded for getting only one answer right.

Each question in this subtest is in the form of either a coded message that you have to decode into English or an English phrase that you have to encode. As the code consists of concepts, it isn't a simple letter-for-letter substitution. This means that there can be a great deal of ambiguity in the decisions that you need to make about which symbols to use and what order to place them in. You can also combine symbols to alter their meaning, which creates further complexity. For example, suppose that you have a symbol for 'hot' and a symbol for 'earth'. Combining the two symbols may mean 'hot earth', but you can also use the combination to describe 'hot sand' or even 'lava'. The Decision Analysis subtest gradually deploys the full scope of this ambiguity, leading to increasingly complex questions as you progress through the subtest.

Unlike some of the other subtests in the UKCAT, this subtest rewards lateral thinking and an ability to apply judgement rather than pure logic to situations.

Doing well in the Decision Analysis subtest

The Decision Analysis subtest rewards good judgement, which generally comes with experience. As the subtest is basically a series of puzzles, doing similar puzzles can enable you to build up experience quickly.

Any puzzle that stretches your ability to think and requires lateral thinking can help you with the Decision Analysis subtest. Riddles are one example, but the most readily available instance is cryptic newspaper crosswords. These crosswords encourage you to think outside the box, drawing on common concepts and conventions to solve the clues. If you already enjoy cryptic crosswords, the Decision Analysis subtest is going to be right up your street.

If you're not a crossword fan, don't worry. There are other ways to improve your ability in this subtest, including creative writing (which encourages the manipulation of ideas and words), thinking about how you make real-life decisions (what facts you use, how you combine the facts and how much weight you give each fact), and practising the sample questions in Chapter 7.

A surprisingly effective way to practise for this subtest is to keep a diary. Human beings are constantly thinking and feeling lots of different things but rarely take time to understand *why* they think and feel those things. Developing insight into your emotions and actions requires you to place some sort of logical framework around those fleeting impulses. This means translating – or decoding – emotional states into concepts, and then encoding those concepts into prose. Ordering the concepts into a narrative structure is the essence of good diary-keeping. Try to make your diary an insightful account of your day, not just a list of events but also the thoughts and feelings that went with them.

Making the right decisions on test day

By the time you get to the Decision Analysis subtest, you'll already be feeling quite tired. Try to cleanse and refresh your mind by following these handy tips:

✔ **Relax for 10 seconds before you start the subtest.** You're under time pressure, but losing 10 seconds isn't the end of the world. Those 10 seconds of relaxation may be just the ticket to refresh yourself. Take a few deep breaths in and out, focus on slowing your breathing and imagine yourself in a happy and relaxed environment.

✔ **Don't be intimidated by the large amount of data at the start of the subtest.** You may see lots of unusual symbols, some annoyingly similar to each other. Simply acknowledge the information and then move on to the test questions.

✔ **Think in concepts, not words.** If you can understand that words and language are merely human constructs applied to underlying concepts, you may find the questions much easier (it helps if you speak a foreign language!). Your job is to fit a round peg into a square hole – just as in real life when you put your thoughts or feelings into words.

✔ **Accept that the questions are deliberately ambiguous.** Feeling some degree of doubt is normal. Don't spend ages going over a question again and again. Keep moving methodically through the subtest – and remember that you have just over a minute per question. You're not expected to get 100%, and nor will anybody else! If something looks really hard, just flag it and return to it later if you have time.

✔ **Remember that the scored parts of the UKCAT are over after you finish this subtest.** Try to summon up the strength to keep going for just a little longer.

Doing the sample questions in Chapter 7 (and other mock questions) can help you deal with the complexity and ambiguity of the actual exam.

Discovering yourself: Situational Judgement subtest

The new-for-2012 Situational Judgement subtest doesn't form part of the application process in 2012 and is included solely for trial purposes. Universities aren't informed of your answers or scores and they don't contribute towards your overall UKCAT score. At the time of writing, no decision has been taken as to whether this subtest is going to become a permanent feature of the UKCAT.

The Situational Judgement subtest is designed to assess personal attributes such as interpersonal skills and ethical values. The question format is a series of hypothetical scenarios based in a clinical setting or during educational training for a medical or dental career. You're asked to read each scenario and make judgements about a series of options in response to it. These responses are then marked against an ideal scoring scheme to provide a picture of your situational judgement. You face 13 scenarios, with 4–6 options to rate, for a total of 60 items.

This subtest consists of two parts. In Part One you rate the *appropriateness* of a series of options in response to the scenario and in Part Two you rate the *importance* of a series of options in response to the scenario.

The Situational Judgement subtest is new and for that reason it's difficult to give lots of advice about it. We can give some general pointers, however, based on our understanding of this ethical test:

- ✔ **Read all scenarios carefully.** Make special note of any areas of risk to you, to other people mentioned in the scenario and to the public.

- ✔ **Think about the impact of each option on you and other people.** For example, in a scenario that requires you to decide on a treatment plan in a situation where the patient, their family, and the doctors all disagree, an option that allows for all parties to come to a negotiated outcome is likely to be better than one where the doctor tries to force his opinion on everyone else.

- ✔ **Don't let your answer to one question affect how you answer the following questions.** Consider each question independently.

- ✔ **Be aware of the limits to your competence.** If an option puts you in a situation that is clearly beyond your competence, it may be unethical to act. For example, if the scenario describes you as a medical student and one of the options requires you to operate on a patient unsupervised, it's probably the wrong answer.

- ✔ **Consider issues from ethical and legal perspectives and try to anticipate what a professional, sensible and compassionate doctor might do.** Whichever option comes closest is probably the correct answer.

A rose by any other name?

The Situational Judgement subtest being trialled in 2012 tests a similar set of attributes (and indeed sounds similar in many respects) to the old non-cognitive analysis section that was removed from the UKCAT in 2011. This subtest aimed to test personal attributes and was, in essence, a form of personality testing designed to assess your suitability to a career in medicine. It was pretty controversial at the time, as many people considered it open to manipulation and unlikely to yield useful information to universities.

We don't doubt that understanding your own personality is very important. Good self-knowledge gives you insight into your interactions with the world around you and how those interactions affect your internal wellbeing. Such insight can help you choose the right career path and lifestyle to maximise your happiness. But trying to assess your personality using a psychometric test before medical school presents real problems. First, misrepresentation is possible, leading to inaccurate results. Second and more fundamentally, many different types of people can have successful medical careers, provided they choose their specialities carefully and have the motivation and ability to cope with those aspects of medical training and practice that don't come to them naturally. The great wartime Prime Minister Sir Winston Churchill would probably have done appallingly in a personality test!

It will be interesting to see whether the new Situational Judgement subtest does a better job than the former non-cognitive analysis subtest. Time will tell.

Chapter 7

Practising the UKCAT

*L*ots of medical schools require that you sit the United Kingdom Clinical Aptitude Test (UKCAT) as part of your application. We list those institutions and describe the test in Chapter 6, but here we provide sample questions for each of the four main subtests in the UKCAT: Verbal Reasoning, Quantitative Reasoning, Abstract Reasoning and Decision Analysis. (We don't supply any for the new Situational Judgement subtest because, at the time of writing, it's only being trialled and doesn't count towards your overall UKCAT score, and may undergo significant changes if and when it's adopted.) Following the questions is a section for the answers, complete with explanations for our reasoning. We suggest that you don't look at the answers until you've tried the questions.

Don't be discouraged if you make mistakes. The whole point of doing sample questions is to prepare yourself for the actual test. Making a few mistakes at this stage means that you're less likely to make them on test day. Also, avoid rushing through this chapter. Time pressure is certainly a significant challenge in the actual exam, but for now concentrate on understanding the answers and doing the best you can, even if that means taking a bit more time than in the real thing. Speed comes with practice and with confidence in your techniques.

This book covers so many aspects of getting into medical school that we don't have space for lots of questions. These sample questions merely serve as a brief introduction to the UKCAT, but you need far more practice than this to be fully prepared for the test. Our companion book *UKCAT For Dummies* (Wiley) has hundreds of questions (including two timed mock tests).

Verbal Reasoning Sample Questions

Read each passage, thinking carefully about the information presented. Use the information to answer each statement. You have to determine whether each statement is true or false, or whether you can't tell.

On test day, you have on average 30 seconds to answer each statement. Don't worry if it takes you longer now; you'll get a lot faster with practice.

Passage 1

Concerning Liberality and Meanness
(Adapted from *The Prince*, by Nicolo Machiavelli)

I say that it would be well to be reputed liberal. Nevertheless, liberality exercised in a way that does not bring you the reputation for it, injures you; for if one exercises it honestly and as it should be exercised, it may not become known, and you will not avoid the reproach of its opposite.

Therefore, anyone wishing to maintain among men the name of liberal is obliged to avoid no attribute of magnificence; so that a prince thus inclined will consume in such acts all his property, and will be compelled in the end, if he wish to maintain the name of liberal, to unduly weigh down his people, and tax them, and do everything he can to get money.

This will soon make him odious to his subjects, and becoming poor he will be little valued by any one; thus, with his liberality, having offended many and rewarded few, he is affected by the very first trouble and imperilled by whatever may be the first danger; recognising this himself, and wishing to draw back from it, he runs at once into the reproach of being miserly.

There is nothing wastes so rapidly as liberality, for even whilst you exercise it you lose the power to do so, and so become either poor or despised, or else, in avoiding poverty, rapacious and hated. And a prince should guard himself, above all things, against being despised and hated; and liberality leads you to both. Therefore, it is wiser to have a reputation for meanness, which brings reproach without hatred, than to be compelled through seeking a reputation for liberality to incur a name for rapacity which begets reproach with hatred.

A – True   B – False   C – Can't tell

Statement 1: According to the author, liberality, if done as it should be, doesn't necessarily result in a person being known for his liberality.

Statement 2: The author believes that long-term liberality in a prince means he spends more money than he has, resulting in tax increases on his population to fund his spending.

Statement 3: The conclusion of the passage is that a reputation for miserliness is more damaging to a prince than a reputation for generosity.

Statement 4: The principles outlined in the passage apply to modern democratic governments.

Passage 2

Rome in Chaos

(Adapted from *The Decline and Fall of the Roman Empire*, by Edward Gibbon)

Pestilence and famine contributed to fill up the measure of the calamities of Rome. The first could be only imputed to the just indignation of the gods; but a monopoly of corn, was considered as the immediate cause of the second. The popular discontent at these calamities, after it had long circulated in whispers, broke out in the assembled circus. The people quitted their favourite amusements for the more delicious pleasure of revenge, rushed in crowds towards a palace in the suburbs, one of the emperor's retirements, and demanded, with angry clamours, the head of the public enemy.

Cleander ordered a body of Praetorian cavalry to sally forth, and disperse the seditious multitude. The multitude fled with precipitation towards the city but when the cavalry entered the streets, their pursuit was checked by a shower of stones and darts from the roofs and windows of the houses. The foot guards, who had been long jealous of the Praetorians, embraced the party of the people. The tumult became a regular engagement. The Praetorians gave way, oppressed with numbers; and the tide of popular fury returned with redoubled violence against the gates of the palace, where the Emperor Commodus lay, dissolved in luxury and alone, unconscious of the civil war.

Commodus started from his dream of pleasure, and commanded that the head of Cleander should be thrown out to the people. The desired spectacle instantly appeased the tumult; and he might even yet have regained the affection and confidence of his subjects.

A – True   B – False   C – Can't tell

Statement 5: A corn monopoly was partially responsible for the outbreak of violence.

Statement 6: Commodus was asleep while the riot was taking place.

Statement 7: The crowd initially routed by cavalry fought back only when the crowd retreated outside the city.

Statement 8: By sacrificing Cleander, Commodus regained the confidence of his subjects.

Passage 3

Creative Thinking and Schizophrenia
(Adapted from *The Meaning of Madness*, by Neel Burton)

At Vanderbilt University, Folley and Park conducted two experiments to compare the creative thinking processes of schizophrenia sufferers, 'schizotypes' (people with traits of schizophrenia), and normal control subjects.

In the first experiment, subjects were asked to make up new functions for household objects. While the schizophrenia sufferers and normal control subjects performed similarly to one another, the schizotypes performed better than either.

In the second experiment, subjects were once again asked to make up new functions for household objects as well as to perform a basic control task while the activity in the prefrontal lobes was monitored by a brain scanning technique called near-infrared optical spectroscopy. While all three groups used both brain hemispheres for creative tasks, the right hemispheres of schizotypes showed hugely increased activation compared to the schizophrenia sufferers and normal controls.

For Folley and Park, these results support their idea that increased use of the right hemisphere and thus increased communication between the brain hemispheres may be related to enhanced creativity in psychosis-prone populations.

A – True   B – False   C – Can't tell

Statement 9: Folley and Park initially assumed that normal controls would perform best in their experiments.

Statement 10: The results of the first experiment were statistically significant.

Statement 11: In the second experiment, the right hemispheres of people with schizophrenia showed increased activation compared with normal controls.

Statement 12: The experiments do not demonstrate that increased communication between the brain hemispheres is related to enhanced creativity in psychosis-prone populations.

Check out the answers to the practice tests later in this chapter.

Quantitative Reasoning Sample Questions

Study each numerical presentation carefully. After each presentation are four questions based on the content within the presentation. Test data in this subtest can be presented in the form of tables, charts and graphs. Your task is to rapidly identify relevant information from the presentation, and then manipulate that information appropriately to answer the question.

On test day, you have on average 38 seconds to answer each question.

Numerical presentation 1

Mental Health Act Assessments (see Table 7-1)

Table 7-1	Distribution of Mental Health Act Assessments in 2010
Month	**Assessments**
January	132
February	85
March	88
April	101
May	95
June	110
July	123
August	117
September	78
October	92
November	167
December	286

Item 1:

How many assessments took place in the first three months of the year?

(A) 132   (B) 217   (C) 305   (D) 318   (E) 406

Item 2:

By the end of which month had 50 per cent of the assessments taken place?

(A) May   (B) Jun   (C) July   (D) August   (E) September

Item 3:

What percentage of assessments, to the nearest whole number, took place in the last three months of the year?

(A) 13%   (B) 21%   (C) 25%   (D) 31%   (E) 37%

Item 4:

The monitoring exercise was repeated in 2011 with the following changes in the numbers of assessments: May (+15), June (–6), July (+7), August (–11). For 2011, what is the ratio of assessments in May and June to those in July and August?

(A) 1:1   (B) 113:129   (C) 41:48   (D) 107:11   (E) 52:65

Numerical presentation 2

Well-heeled

James is just starting his career and decides to buy three pairs of shoes to suit any basic professional need (black plain cap-toe oxfords, dark brown wingtip oxfords and burgundy penny loafers).

He's undecided whether to buy high-quality but expensive Northampton Classics or cheaper but limited-lifespan Mass Markets and so draws up Tables 7-2 and 7-3 to compare the costs and help reach a decision.

Table 7-2	Northampton Classics
Pair of shoes	£650
Factory recrafting and resoling (required every 5 years; can be done a maximum of 3 times per shoe)	£120 per pair
High-quality polish (total annual cost)	£20
Lasted shoe trees (pair)	£50
Expected lifetime, with good upkeep	20 years per pair

Table 7-3	Mass Markets
Pair of shoes	£75
Cheap polish (total annual cost)	£5
Cheap shoe trees (pair)	£10
Expected lifetime, with good upkeep	2 years per pair

Item 5:

How much would it cost James to wear Northampton Classics over a 40-year career, assuming he can reuse the old shoe trees in any new pairs of shoes he needs to buy over that career?

(A) £5,060 (B) £6,210   (C) £7,010   (D) £7,160 (E) £7,730

Item 6:

How much would it cost him to wear Mass Markets over the same career? (Assume the cheaper shoe trees break and need to be repurchased once every 20 years.)

(A) £1,760 (B) £4,560   (C) £4,565   (D) £4,730 (E) £4,760

Item 7:

Which of the following statements is false?

A – Northampton Classics are more expensive over a career lifetime than Mass Markets.

B – If cost is the only determinant of purchase, James should buy Mass Markets.

C – If James finds the aesthetic value and craftsmanship of Northampton Classics to be superior to that of Mass Markets, he may find them worth spending extra money on.

D – The annual cost of wearing Northampton Classics is £175.25.

E – The annual cost of wearing Mass Markets is £110.00.

Item 8:

James decides to buy Northampton Classics, but starts off with four pairs of shoes instead of three, and for that fourth pair adds dark brown Chelsea boots to his collection. This addition reduces the wear on each pair of shoes and so reduces the required frequency of resoling. Assuming that resoling is the limiting factor in determining the lifespan of the shoe, how many years will each pair now last him?

(A) 22.5   (B) 24.3   (C) 25.5   (D) 26.7   (E) 30.3

Numerical presentation 3

Eating into the market

Figure 7-1 shows the changing market shares of three major UK supermarkets.

Item 9:

In 1997, what's the approximate ratio of Blue Skies' market share to that of Big Green?

(A) 3:2   (B) 9:5   (C) 17:10   (D) 19:10   (E) 2:1

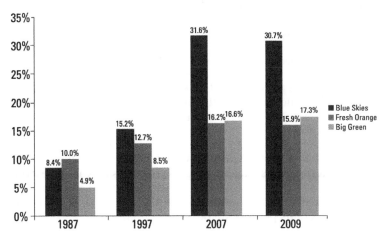

Figure 7-1: Evolving supermarket market shares over the years.

Item 10:

Which of the following statements is supported by the information in the chart?

A – Blue Skies' market share is steadily increasing.

B – Big Green's market share is steadily falling.

C – The three supermarkets in the chart have taken an ever-increasing share of the overall market.

D – The combined market share of the three supermarkets suffered a fall in 2009.

E – Discount grocers are responsible for Blue Skies' market share fall in 2009 relative to 2007.

Item 11:

Total grocery sales in the UK are approximately £125 billion per year. Roughly how much of that did Big Green take in 2009?

(A) £6.1 billion   (B) £10.6 billion   (C) £20.8 billion
(D) £21.6 billion   (E) £38.4 billion

Item 12:

What's the range in market share between the three supermarkets in 1997?

(A) 6.7%   (B) 14.8%   (C) 15.0%   (D) 15.4%   (E) 26.7%

Abstract Reasoning Sample Questions

Study the pairs of sets in the displays in Figures 7-2, 7-3 and 7-4. All the shapes within a set share a similarity, which distinguishes them from the shapes in the other set of the pair.

You're presented with a series of five questions for each display. The questions take the form of a new test shape. Your task is to determine whether the test shape belongs to Set A, Set B or neither set.

The subtest assesses how you infer relationships from the patterns of abstract shapes. The patterns may include irrelevant and distracting material that either obscures the real relationship or presents a red herring. In the UKCAT, you'll have an average of 15 seconds per test shape.

Display 1

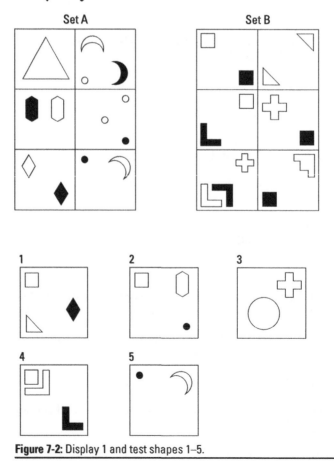

Figure 7-2: Display 1 and test shapes 1–5.

Display 2

Set A   Set B

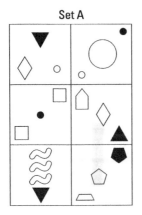 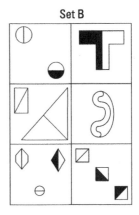

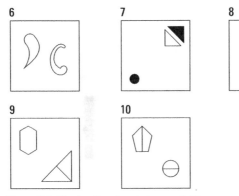

Figure 7-3: Display 2 and test shapes 6–10.

Display 3

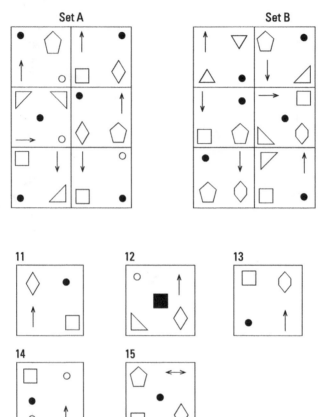

Figure 7-4: Display 3 and test shapes 11–15.

Decision Analysis Sample Questions

Read the scenario and study the code provided in Table 7-4. The questions then ask you to either encode or decode a message using the code, or to decide upon additions to the code. The UKCAT test provides approximately 74 seconds per question in this subtest.

Unlike questions in the other subtests, Decision Analysis questions have four or five response options, and more than one answer may be correct. The question states whether you need to select more than one answer.

Scenario

The Turin Codex

Legend tells of a mysterious and powerful organisation called The Penumbra Syndicate responsible for influencing world history down through the ages. Syndicate members are said to communicate with each other through a strange system of codes, but little progress was made in understanding this until the dazzling recent archaeological discovery of The Turin Codex, which reveals the symbolic basis for at least part of the code (see Table 7-4).

Table 7-4		The Turin Codex	
Nouns	**Verbs**	**Adjectives**	**Operators**
I = ○	Kill = ☄	Rich = ✿	Positive = ♪
You = ●	Talk = ▥	Poor = ✹	Negative = ℗
He = ■	Pay = ✉	Angry = ☹	Quickly = ☞
King = ♈	Run = ♉	Calm = ☺	Slowly = ☜
Pope = ♱	Sail = ♒	Brave = ♢	Now = ♌
Queen = ♍	Ride = ♐	Cowardly = ♦	Then = ⚡
Cardinal = ♎	Take = ❽		Conditional = ♎
Knight = ♞	Burn = ♋		
Peasant = ♦			
Home = ❖			

Armed with the Codex, your task is to decipher the following messages written in the Penumbra Syndicate's code, convert some others into Penumbra code and thereby save the world from their malign and pervasive influence!

Question 1

What is the best interpretation of the following Penumbra message?

♎, ⚡☄, ♈

A – The king will be killed by the cardinal

B – The cardinal has killed the king

C – The cardinal will be killed by the king

D – The king has talked to the cardinal

E – The king might kill the cardinal

Question 2

What is the best interpretation of the following Penumbra message?

$$(\mathbf{O}\bullet)(\aleph\wp), \, \Omega(\mathbf{O}, \bullet, \blacksquare)$$

A – I'm trapped – you have to get help now!

B – We're trapped – call for back-up immediately!

C – We're trapped; it's now every man for himself!

D – Don't move – I'll come to help you

E – We must all remain perfectly still

Question 3

The Turin Codex is an incomplete portion of modern Penumbra Syndicate code. In particular, the code has been added to over the centuries to include symbols for things that simply weren't in existence at the time the Codex was laid down. Which two of the following would be the most useful additions to Syndicate code if attempting to convey the following message?

> *Modern politicians need to use the Internet, television and road tours to communicate effectively with their people.*

A – Politician

B – Internet

C – Television

D – Road tours

E – Communicate

Checking Your Answers

In this section we supply the answers and explanations to the UKCAT sample questions from the preceding section.

Verbal Reasoning subtest

Passage 1

Answer 1

A – True

The passage is quite dense, with many subordinate clauses, which makes it challenging to read and to extract information. The first paragraph includes the lengthy sentence 'Nevertheless, liberality exercised in a way that does not bring you the reputation for it, injures you; for if one exercises it honestly and as it should be exercised, it may not become known, and you will not avoid the reproach of its opposite.'

By removing clauses irrelevant to the statement under scrutiny, you can reduce this statement to 'Liberality, if one exercises it honestly as it should be, may not become known'. Therefore the statement is true.

Although you don't need to know this to answer the question, 'liberality' in this context refers to spending vast quantities of money, especially on public enterprises.

Answer 2

A – True

The relevant information is in the second paragraph:

> . . . *anyone wishing to maintain among men the name of liberal is obliged to avoid no attribute of magnificence; so that a prince thus inclined will consume in such acts all his property, and will be compelled in the end, if he wish to maintain the name of liberal, to unduly weigh down his people, and tax them, and do everything he can to get money.*

You can simplify this logically to 'Anyone trying to maintain a liberal reputation is inclined to consume all his property, and to tax his people to get money.' It then becomes obvious that the statement is true.

Answer 3

B – False

According to the passage, the opposite is true. The passage suggests that liberality eventually results in people hating the prince and considering him wrong. Being miserly also results in people considering the prince wrong, but because tax rises haven't been required the people don't hate the prince as well.

Therefore being liberal causes more damage to the prince's reputation than being miserly.

Answer 4

C – Can't tell

The passage, unsurprisingly for one written during the Italian Renaissance, draws no parallels with modern democratic government. Although you can theorise that the same basic principles of wise economic management apply to the popularity of an elected government as much as they did to Florentine nobility, you can't state this for certain based solely on the information provided in the passage.

Passage 2

Answer 5

A – True

To the population of Rome, the corn monopoly 'was considered the immediate cause' of the famine. The famine, alongside pestilence (disease), was one of the 'calamities of Rome' that led to the 'popular discontent' that culminated in the violent scenes alluded to in the passage. The passage therefore describes a logical sequence starting with the corn monopoly and ending in violence.

You don't need to know whether the corn monopoly was actually the cause of the famine in order to determine the statement's veracity – you simply need to know that the Romans considered this to be true. The Romans may or may not have been right to do so.

Answer 6

A – True

The passage describes Commodus as waking from a 'dream of pleasure' and being previously unconscious of the civil war. Therefore Commodus was asleep when these events took place.

Answer 7

B – False

The passage says that missiles thrown from houses on the streets checked the pursuit of the Praetorian cavalry. Therefore the crowd didn't retreat outside the city but fought the Praetorians from within the city.

Answer 8

C – Can't tell

The passage only says that he 'might even have regained . . . the confidence of his subjects', not that he did so. You still don't know the actual eventual outcome by the end of the passage.

Passage 3

Answer 9

B – False

The last paragraph of the passage states that '*For Folley and Park*', the results of the experiments 'support *their* idea that increased use of the right hemisphere and thus increased communication between the brain hemispheres may be related to *enhanced* creativity in psychosis-prone populations.' This means that they didn't originally assume that normal controls would perform best. They assumed that the psychosis-prone populations would perform better than the controls.

You don't need to know whether Folley and Park's initial assumption was that schizotypes would outperform schizophrenics (and, indeed, you can't logically derive this information from the text). You need to know only that Folley and Park thought normal controls would have been outperformed.

The statement requires you to separate out the descriptive portions of the passage from those where the author describes Folley and Park's own position.

Answer 10

C – Can't tell

The text states that the schizotypes performed better than the people with schizophrenia and normal control subjects. However, the text doesn't specify how much better, the sample size or any derived statistics. Statements regarding significance are therefore impossible to verify or disprove.

Answer 11

C – Can't tell

The passage says that the right hemispheres of the schizotypes showed hugely increased activation compared with the people with schizophrenia and normal controls. However, the text doesn't specify which of the people with schizophrenia and normal controls showed higher activation.

Although the answer to this question would almost certainly be present in the full results of the experiment, the answer isn't available in the text provided.

Answer 12

A – True

The text says that, even for Folley and Park, the results *support the idea* that increased use of the right hemisphere and thus increased communication between the brain hemispheres may be related to enhanced creativity in psychosis-prone populations.

This question is a reminder not to over-interpret the passage.

If the experiment's results didn't provide even the experimenters with enough confidence to assert this statement's veracity such that they merely couch it as 'supporting' the idea, you certainly can't draw such a firm conclusion solely from the information provided in the passage.

You may be tempted to assume that the experiment's results are valid and universal, but the passage certainly doesn't imply as much.

Quantitative Reasoning subtest

Numerical Presentation 1

Answer 1

C – 305

This test is a straightforward check of your ability to extract the relevant data from the table and then add the data together to find the total. The relevant data for the answer is included in Table 7-5.

Table 7-5	Assessments in the First Three Months
Month	**Assessments**
January	132
February	85
March	88

The sum of 132, 85 and 88 is 305.

Answer 2

D – August

This problem is a two-step operation. First you need to find 50 per cent of the total number of assessments. The total is 1,474 (calculated by adding up each of the individual data points). The 50 per cent mark is therefore 737 assessments.

Then work your way down the table, adding up the assessments as you go, until you go past 737. This occurs after you pass August, so the answer is D.

Answer 3

E – 37%

First you need to find the total number of assessments that took place in the last three months of the year, as per Table 7-6.

The total is 92 + 167 + 286 = 545.

As the total number of assessments is 1,474 (which you already calculated for Answer 2), the percentage is 545 ÷ 1,474 × 100 = 37 per cent to the nearest whole number.

Table 7-6	Assessments in the Last Three Months
Month	**Assessments**
October	92
November	167
December	286

Answer 4

D – 107:118

You've been given the changes with respect to the original (2010) data. You can quickly determine the new totals, as outlined in Table 7-7.

Table 7-7	New Distribution of Assessments in 2011
Month	**Assessments**
May	95 + 15 = 110
June	110 – 6 = 104
July	123 + 7 = 130
August	117 – 11 = 106

To work out the ratio between the months of May and June, and July and August, you need to add up the relevant data points:

> May + June = 110 + 104 = 214
>
> July + August = 130 + 106 = 236

The ratio 214:236 simplifies to 107:118.

Numerical Presentation 2

Answer 5

C – £7,010

Each pair of Northampton Classics lasts 20 years. James has a 40-year career, and so he needs two pairs of each of the three types of shoe he wants to buy, making a total requirement of six pairs. The shoe cost is therefore £650 × 6 = £3,900.

He needs to resole each pair three times during its 20-year lifespan, giving a total of (6 × 3) = 18 resoles. The resoling cost is £120 × 18 = £2,160.

The polish costs are £20 × 40 years = £800.

As he can reuse them, James needs only three pairs of shoe trees. Tree costs are £50 × 3 = £150.

The total cost for wearing Northampton Classics over 40 years is therefore (£3,900 + £2,160 + £800 + £150) = £7,010.

Answer 6

E – £4,760

James needs 20 pairs of each type of shoe, making a total of (20 × 3) = 60 pairs. The total shoe cost is therefore 60 × £75 = £4,500.

The shoe polish costs are £5 × 40 = £200.

As they last only 20 years, James needs six pairs of shoe trees, resulting in a tree cost of 6 × £10 = £60.

The total cost of wearing Mass Markets is therefore (£4,500 + £200 + £60) = £4,760.

Answer 7

E – The annual cost of wearing Mass Markets is £110

This is false. The actual cost is £4,760 ÷ 40 = £119.

All the other statements are true.

Answer 8

D – 26.7

The new resoling interval is proportionally increased to 4 ÷ 3 × 5 years = 6.67 years.

James can still resole each pair of shoes three times, meaning the shoes now last 6.67 + (6.67 × 3) = 26.7 years (approximately).

Alternatively, you can simply multiply the initial 20-year lifespan figure by 4 ÷ 3.

Numerical Presentation 3

Answer 9

B – 9.5

In 1997, Blue Skies took 15.7 per cent of the market and Big Green took 8.5 per cent. The ratio between the two is 15.7:8.5, or approximately 1.8:1, which is equivalent to 9:5.

Answer 10

D – The combined market share of the three supermarkets suffered a fall in 2009

Options A-C are demonstrably false. Option E cannot be verified on the basis of the information in the chart.

Answer 11
D – £21.6 billion

125 billion × 17.3% = £21.6 billion

Answer 12
A – 6.7%

In 1997, the greatest market share was Blue Skies with 15.2 per cent and the smallest market share was Big Green with 8.5 per cent. The range is therefore (15.2 – 8.5) = 6.7%.

Abstract Reasoning subtest

Display 1
1. Neither set; **2.** Neither set; **3.** Neither set; **4.** Set B; **5.** Set A

All the examples in Set A contain items with no right angles. All the examples in Set B contain items with at least one right angle. The exact nature of the overall shape, the colour and the orientation show no consistent features of commonality.

Test shapes 1, 2 and 3 have objects both with and without right angles and so aren't Set A or Set B. Test shape 4 has only right-angled figures and so belongs to Set B. Test shape 5 contains objects with no right angles and so belongs to Set A.

Display 2
6. Set A; **7.** Set A; **8.** Set A; **9.** Neither set; **10.** Set B

Set A's objects are undivided. Set B's objects are subdivided.

Test shapes 6, 7 and 8 contain objects without subdivision and so belong in Set A. Test shape 9 has a mixture of whole and divided objects and so isn't in Set A or Set B. Test shape 10 has subdivided objects and so is part of Set B.

Display 3
11. Set A; **12.** Neither set; **13.** Set B; **14.** Neither set; **15.** Neither set

The black circle is the key to these sets. In Set A, if the black circle is at the top of the shape, the arrow points up. If the black circle is in the middle, the arrow is horizontal. If the black circle is at the bottom, the arrow points down. In Set B, the top/bottom rule is reversed but the middle rule remains the same.

Test shape 11 obeys Set A's rules. Test shape 12 has no black circle and so belongs to neither set. Test shape 13 obeys Set

B's rules. Test shapes 14 and 15 fall into neither set because the arrows don't obey the rules of either set.

Decision Analysis subtest

Answer 1

A – The king will be killed by the cardinal

♤, ⧖◉※, ↝

= Cardinal, Then Kill, King

= Cardinal, kill at some point in the future, king = The king will be killed by the cardinal

You can't express the future perfect tense using the Turin Codex, but this answer is as close as you can get. In any case, no other option quite fits the code.

Answer 2

C – We're trapped; it's now every man for himself!

(◉●)(♉♟), ♌(◉,●, ■)

= (I You)(Run Negative), Now (I, You, He)

= We (can't run), it's now all of us separate

= We're trapped; it's now every man for himself!

Answer 3

B – Internet   and   C – Television

You can encode the word 'Politician' with 'Talk Knight' or 'Talk Peasant', depending on your level of respect for politicians. The term 'Road Tours' can be 'Ride Quickly' – or even 'Ride Quickly, Peasant Peasant Home' if you want to convey a sense of visiting the electorate. You can convey 'Communicate' with 'Talk'.

On the other hand, conveying 'Internet' or 'Television' without some new code is much harder.

Chapter 8

Breaking Down the BMAT

*A*s part of their selection procedure, certain universities require applicants to sit the Bio-Medical Admissions Test (BMAT), which is a test designed to stretch even the most capable students.

In this chapter we discuss the BMAT in detail and lead you through preparing for it.

Grasping the Purpose of the BMAT

The BMAT is a test of academic ability. It rewards the most academically gifted candidates through a rigorous series of multiple choice and short answer questions that test generic skills and knowledge of scientific topics. It also incorporates an essay section.

Cambridge Assessments developed the BMAT specifically in response to concerns raised by some of the top medical and veterinary schools. They'd lost confidence in A-level grades as an adequate predictor of subsequent success at medical and veterinary school. As a result, they pushed for an alternative, more rigorous entrance exam.

The BMAT is designed to be highly challenging in order to differentiate between students at the top end of the academic scale.

Sitting the BMAT

You're asked to sit the BMAT when you apply to certain medical or veterinary schools. The test is a required part of the selection process for the medical courses and universities listed in Table 8-1. In Table 8-2, we explain what the UCAS (Universities and Colleges Admissions Service) course codes used in Table 8-1 mean.

Table 8-1	Universities and Courses Requiring the BMAT
University	*UCAS Course Code*
Imperial College London	A100, B900, B9N2
Cambridge	A100, A101 (not compulsory), D100
University College London	A100
Oxford	A100, A101, BC98
The Royal Veterinary College	D100, D101, D102

Table 8-2	UCAS Course Codes
UCAS Code	*Course*
A100	Medicine
A101	Medicine (graduate entry 4-year programme)
B900	Biomedical Sciences
B9N2	Biomedical Sciences with Management
BC98	Biomedical Sciences. BA (Hons) is awarded in either Cell and Systems Biology or Neuroscience
D100	Veterinary Medicine
D101	BSc/BVetMed Combined Degree
D102	Graduate Accelerated BVetMed

Therefore, for undergraduate medical school applicants, the BMAT is required by Cambridge, Imperial, Oxford and UCL.

Cambridge University suggests that graduate applicants sit the BMAT, specifying that a good score is looked upon favourably during the selection process; however, sitting the exam is not technically mandatory. If you're likely to do well on the BMAT (and most applicants to Cambridge fall into this category), we advise that you give it a shot.

As of the 2012 cycle (i.e. for 2013 entry), Oxford requires graduate medical applicants to sit the BMAT rather than the UKCAT (see Chapters 6 and 7). This is a change from previous years, and brings Oxford's graduate entry requirements into closer alignment with the undergraduate course.

Knowing the important dates

You can't defer your BMAT scores to subsequent years, which means that you have to sit the exam in the autumn of the year of your application.

The exact dates for the BMAT registration, testing and publication of results cycle vary annually, usually by not more than a few days. The BMAT's website contains all the relevant dates for the current year. You can find it at www.admissionstests.cambridge assessment.org.uk/adt/bmat and it contains lots of other useful information too. Table 8-3 lists the dates for a typical cycle.

Table 8-3	Key BMAT Dates for a Typical Cycle
Event	*Date*
Registration opens	1 September
Standard entry closing date	1 October
Last date for entry (late fees apply)	15 October
Last date for reimbursement of fees	15 October
Test date	7 November
Results day	21 November
Last date for results enquiry submissions	28 November

You don't have a choice about the test date. Plan ahead and clear your diary for the week leading up to the exam.

If your medical school choices mean that you also need to take the UKCAT (which we describe in Chapters 6 and 7), we recommend sitting the UKCAT earlier in the cycle. The UKCAT's final test dates tend to be in the first week of October; this would leave you less than a month to focus exclusively on the BMAT, which, in light of all your other commitments, we feel is much too short.

Although revision for the UKCAT can help towards the BMAT, we believe that allowing a gap of a couple of months makes the overall process easier.

You can get your fees reimbursed if you need to cancel your test, as long as you do so before the cancellation deadline (indicated in Table 8-3).

Considering the registration process

The BMAT registration is processed through an approved BMAT centre. Two types of centre exist:

- ✔ **Closed centres** only accept applications from pupils studying at that centre. Many schools and further education colleges fall into this category.

- ✔ **Open centres** accept outside applicants too. If your school or college isn't a closed centre, find your nearest open centre via the search engine at www.admissionstests.cambridge assessment.org.uk/adt/findcentre.

As the search engine demonstrates, the BMAT can be sat all around the world. Over 6,000 candidates across nearly 100 countries sit the test.

The BMAT entry fee is £42.50 provided you register for the test before the standard entry closing date (shown for 2012 in Table 8-3). After that, you can still register provided you submit your application before the last date for entry and pay an extra £30 in late fees. Non-EU candidates pay that total of £72.50 regardless of when they register.

You can get your standard entry fees reimbursed if you receive certain grants or awards. In the UK, these were traditionally a full Adult Learning Grant (ALG), a full Maintenance Grant, Income-Based Job Seeker's Allowance or Income Support. Recent changes to the benefits system have led to the closure or modification of some of these payments and the organisers haven't as yet clarified how these changes are going to affect the BMAT's reimbursement procedures.

Candidates who believe that they qualify for reimbursement should talk to their school or, if they are sitting the test at an open centre, to BMAT directly. If you do write to BMAT, make sure to enclose a photocopy of proof of entitlement. The postal address that you're going to need is: BMAT Support Team, Cambridge Assessment, 1 Hills Road, Cambridge CB1 2EU, United Kingdom.

Individual centres have the discretion to impose additional charges that can't be reimbursed.

Allowances can be made for candidates who produce written clinical evidence of special educational needs, or other disabilities that impair their ability to complete the test in the allotted time. If you're in such a position, make sure to discuss this with your test centre well in advance of the test date.

Facing test day with confidence

Make sure that you know where you're going on test day! The test starts promptly at 9 a.m. so be sure to take rush-hour traffic into account when setting off on your journey. You need to go through some formalities before sitting the exam, so arrive about half an hour early.

If you're going to an open centre, carry photographic proof of identity such as a valid adult passport or a photocard driving licence. If you have neither of these, ask your school to provide you with a certified letter.

You also need to bring a pencil, an eraser and a black ink pen; some test centres do provide these items, but you can't depend on it. Anyway, you'll probably feel more at ease using your own equipment. You're not permitted to take anything else into the test room, not even your mobile phone.

You aren't allowed to use a calculator.

Inside the test room, you're given a Statement of Entry, which includes a Candidate Number beginning with the letter B followed by five digits. You need to write this number on all exam scripts. You also need to include the Candidate Number of your UCAS form, so that the universities you've applied to can access your results. Cambridge applicants need to omit the starting letter B when including it on the separate Cambridge Application Form.

The Statement of Entry also includes a PIN code, which you use together with your Candidate Number to access your results.

BMAT results are published online at `https://results.cambridgeassessment.org.uk/candidates/controller/open/login.html` on results day. You need to register for access ahead of time (flip to the earlier 'Considering the registration process' section for further details).

Universities access your results directly and can also see your essay. For this reason don't write anything so unreasonable or controversial that it raises concerns about your suitability to become a doctor!

Working efficiently on test day

The BMAT is a challenging exam with intense time pressure. The following hints are designed to help you retain focus (for more detailed information, check out 'Examining the test's sections' later in this chapter):

- ✔ **Read all questions quickly but carefully.**

- ✔ **Avoid skim reading, especially on the Aptitude and Skills section.** It can result in unwarranted assumptions and careless errors.

- ✔ **Don't be intimidated by questions in the Aptitude and Skills section or the Writing Task on unfamiliar topics.** Testers want to know how well you can manipulate numerical information and think about concepts, not whether you're familiar with the subject matter itself.

- ✔ **Write legibly so that examiners can read what you write.** If you have poor penmanship, practise writing short essays under a time constraint. If your writing is really awful, consider printing your letters.

- ✔ **Don't overcomplicate.** If you find yourself drawing on A-level knowledge in the Scientific Knowledge and Applications section, you're probably overcomplicating the question and heading down the wrong track.

- ✔ **Don't spend too much time on questions you can't answer.** Move on to the next question and stay relaxed.

- ✔ **Accept that this exam is tough.** Just focus on doing your best!

Analysing the BMAT's Structure

The BMAT is a pen, pencil and paper exam that lasts two hours. The test consists of three parts: Aptitude and Skills, Scientific Knowledge and Applications, and the Writing Task.

Each of the three parts is independently timed. The Aptitude and Skills, and Scientific Knowledge and Applications sections are a blend of multiple choice and short answer questions, whereas the Writing Task calls for an essay that is no longer than one side of A4 (or, if you have special needs that enable you to use a laptop, 550 words).

Examining the test's sections

Here we take you through each of the sections in detail so that you know what to revise and to avoid nasty surprises.

Aptitude and Skills

This section tests generic skills often used in undergraduate study, including:

- ✔ **Problem solving:** The ability to use numerical information to solve problems. This section checks that you can select relevant information, recognise similar cases and decide on the procedure to apply to arrive at the correct answer.

- ✔ **Understanding argument:** The ability to read information and identify assumptions and flaws, and to distil meaning and arrive at the appropriate conclusions.

- ✔ **Data analysis and inference:** The ability to interpret and manipulate verbal, statistical and graphical sources of data.

Many of the techniques we suggest in Chapter 6 for preparing for the Verbal Reasoning and Quantitative Reasoning subtests of the UKCAT also apply to preparing for the Aptitude and Skills section of the BMAT. The format of the questions does differ, however, so do check out the BMAT questions we provide in Chapter 9 as well.

Scientific Knowledge and Applications

This section is based on the National Curriculum Key Stage 4 (essentially GCSE) standard of Biology, Chemistry, Physics and Mathematics. But it frequently stretches that knowledge or requires you to use it in unusual or imaginative ways.

By the time you sit the BMAT, you're well into your A-level studies. You may be tempted to use this advanced knowledge to solve difficult BMAT problems, especially those in Physics and Mathematics, but we suggest you don't. The BMAT questions are designed to test GCSE level knowledge only. If you think you have to use A-level content, you've probably missed the point of the question.

If you're not currently studying one of the science or maths subjects tested in the BMAT, revise it up to GCSE level to refresh your memory. You don't need any of the botanical elements of Biology, the geological/environmental sciences parts of Chemistry or the seismology bits of Physics.

You can get a flavour of the questions in the Scientific Knowledge and Applications section of the BMAT in Chapter 9.

Writing Task

This section tests your ability to reason around a topic and express your thoughts cogently. It offers you a choice of four questions, and you can choose to answer any one of the four. The questions span topics across general, scientific, veterinary and medical topics. They usually take the form of a *proposition* (a statement) and ask you to discuss its meaning, implications, counter-arguments and potential impact.

Of course you can't research every topic that may come up on the Writing Task, but keeping up to date with healthcare issues occasionally pays off. So the suggestions made in Chapter 4 for keeping up to date with the world of medicine are also relevant here.

Even if you've never even considered your chosen topic before, you should be able to write a strong essay. The exam format gives you a skeleton framework for discussing the topic. To flesh out that framework, you must draw on logic and general knowledge. Think laterally and creatively: think about related topics and illustrate your arguments with striking or original examples.

You can tackle questions involving an ethical dilemma by thinking sequentially about its impact on areas such as financials, health, personal happiness, state and/or societal needs and benefits, and so on. Explore such domains and weigh them up to reach a balanced conclusion.

Practise summarising the debates around controversial topics to get you into the habit of exploring a topic from all angles. You only have one side of A4, so plan your essay carefully beforehand and be accurate and concise.

The Writing Task also assesses the quality of your written English. Revise the basic elements of grammar, style and punctuation. Check out useful style guides at www.economist.com/style guide/introduction and www.bbc.co.uk/journalism/skills/writing).

The good and scrupulous writer

George Orwell once wrote of the scrupulous writer: 'In every sentence that he writes, will ask himself at least four questions, thus: What am I trying to say? What words will express it? What image or idiom will make it clearer? Is this image fresh enough to have an effect? And he will probably ask himself two more: Could I put it more shortly? Have I said anything that is avoidably ugly?'

Mark Twain described how good writers treat sentences: 'At times he may indulge himself with a long one, but he will make sure there are no folds in it, no vaguenesses, no parenthetical interruptions of its view as a whole; when he has done with it, it won't be a sea-serpent with half of its arches under the water; it will be a torch-light procession.'

Take the advice of these two expert novelists to heart!

Chapter 9 contains a sample Writing Task question, together with a model answer and an explanation of why it would receive a very high score.

Getting your timing right

The time pressure in the BMAT is intense. For each section of the test, Table 8-4 lists the time allowed, the number of questions and the resulting time per question.

Table 8-4	Timings for the BMAT Sections		
Section	*Time Allowed*	*Questions*	*Time per Question*
Aptitude and Skills	60 minutes	35 items	Approximately 103 seconds
Scientific Knowledge and Applications	30 minutes	27 items	Approximately 67 seconds
Writing Task	30 minutes	1 from a choice of 4	30 minutes

The timings give you a general idea of how to pace yourself through each section, though naturally some questions are harder than others and may require a little longer. But then remember to be quicker with the simpler ones. There will probably be some questions that you simply won't be able to answer. Don't waste your precious time on those: just come back to them later if you have time; if you don't, just make an educated guess at the answer. The real challenge is in fact the time pressure. So you need to think and act strategically.

Specimen tests and past papers are available at www.admissions tests.cambridgeassessment.org.uk/adt/bmat/Test+ Preparation). We strongly recommend that you go through these questions, as well as going through Chapter 9 in this book.

Making sure you understand the marking

The first two sections of the BMAT (Aptitude and Skills, and Scientific Knowledge and Applications) are marked according to the number of correct responses. There is no *negative marking*, which means that your score doesn't suffer if you guess wrongly. Bottom line is: always put down an answer.

Table 8-5 indicates the distribution of marks for the Aptitude and Skills section.

Table 8-5   Aptitude and Skills Marking Scheme

Domain Being Tested	Approximate Time per Domain (minutes)	Marks Available
Problem solving	30	13
Understanding argument	15	10
Data analysis and inference	15	12

The distribution of marks for the Scientific Knowledge and Applications section is indicated in Table 8-6.

**Table 8-6   Scientific Knowledge and Applications
Marking Scheme**

Domain Being Tested	Approximate Time per Domain (minutes)	Marks Available
Biology	8	6–8
Chemistry	8	6–8
Physics	8	6–8
Mathematics	6	5–7

Your marks for Sections 1 and 2 are independently scaled and cali-brated to give a score on the *BMAT scale,* which runs from 1 (low) to 9 (high). Scores are reported with an accuracy of one decimal place. The distribution of scores is normal. Extreme scores are rare and typical applicants score around 5.0. The best applicants score better, but 6.0 represents a comparatively high score and only exceptional applicants achieve scores in excess of 7.0.

Most students sitting the BMAT have never sat an exam with such a low average score and you may find it disconcerting to receive that kind of score. But do bear in mind that everyone else taking the test is in the same boat.

The Writing Task is marked differently. You're marked indepen-dently on the quality of your content and the quality of your English. However, if the quality of your English is very poor, your content is going to be very difficult to decipher.

Quality of Content is scored from 0 to 5, with 5 being the maximum:

- ✔ **Score 0** is awarded to irrelevant, trivial, unintelligible or miss-ing answers. You have to answer the question in order to score points; correct but irrelevant information doesn't earn you credit.

- ✔ **Score 1** is given to answers that have some bearing on the question but which don't address the question in the way demanded, or are incoherent or unfocused.

- ✔ **Score 2** means that most of the components of the question are answered in a reasonably logical way. Significant elements of confusion in the argument may be present and you may misconstrue certain important aspects of the main propo-sition or its implication, or may provide an unconvincing counter-proposition.

- ✔ **Score 3** is the typical score. It indicates a reasonably well-argued answer that addresses all aspects of the question, making reasonable use of the material provided and generating a reasonable counter-proposition. The argument is relatively rational. Some weakness may exist in the force of the argument or the coherence of the ideas, or some aspect of the argument may have been overlooked.

- ✔ **Score 4** is awarded to good answers with few weaknesses. All aspects of the question are addressed, with good use of the material and generating a good counter-proposition or argument. The argument is rational. Ideas are expressed and arranged in a coherent way, with a balanced consideration of the proposition and counter-proposition.

- ✔ **Score 5** is given only to excellent answers with no significant weaknesses. All aspects of the question are addressed, making great use of the material and generating an outstanding counter-proposition or argument. The argument is cogent. Ideas are expressed in a clear and logical way, considering a breadth of relevant points and leading to a compelling synthesis or conclusion.

Quality of English is scored from A to E:

- ✔ **Band A** essays demonstrate fluent use of English with good sentence structure, vocabulary, grammar, spelling and punctuation.

- ✔ **Band C** essays are reasonably fluent with simple sentence structure and fair grammar. Spelling is reasonable and vocabulary appropriate.

- ✔ **Band E** essays show poor use of English. Sentences are difficult to follow, with grammar and spelling errors. Vocabulary is poor and paragraphing weak.

- ✔ **X** is scored for a shockingly poor use of English.

A typical essay scores around 3A.

Using the test scores

Each university decides for itself how it uses the BMAT in its selection procedure, although all give it very significant weight.

Universities don't consistently reveal the details of their weighing-up process. In our experience, a very good BMAT score (one placing you in the top third of candidates) almost certainly gets you an interview provided, of course, that you meet the other entry criteria.

Oxford and Cambridge demand slightly higher BMAT scores than Imperial and UCL, but even these demand fairly high scores.

If you don't do so well on the BMAT, just put it behind you and do your best, focusing especially on those universities that don't require it.

Chapter 9

Studying BMAT Questions and Answers

In This Chapter

▶ Trying out some BMAT questions

▶ Analysing great answers

*A*s we describe in Chapter 8, some medical schools require you to sit the Bio-Medical Admissions Test (BMAT). To help your preparation, we provide sample questions for each of the BMAT's three sections: Aptitude and Skills, Scientific Knowledge and Applications, and the Writing Task. We also supply answers together with detailed explanations: make sure you read these *after* you've tried the questions yourself.

Making mistakes while tackling these questions is fine, because the aim at this point is to prepare you for the actual test. Besides, discovering that you made a mistake here means that you're far less likely to repeat it on test day.

Take your time with the questions. Don't worry about the time pressures of the actual test, just focus on understanding what the questions require. As you build up your confidence, you'll naturally gain speed.

The BMAT is a tough exam. You'll need to practise many more questions than we've room to provide in this book, which covers every aspect of the application process. More practice tests can be found on the BMAT's website, and there are also commercially available books and preparation courses.

Aptitude and Skills Sample Questions

This section tests generic skills that are required for undergraduate study, including problem solving, understanding argument, and data analysis and inference. In the exam, you have approximately 103 seconds per question.

Question 1

Which two of these statements are analogous?

A. Cassandra is less to be believed than Jonah.

B. Jonah is not more to be believed than Cassandra.

C. Jonah is neither more nor less to be believed as Cassandra.

D. Cassandra is at least as much to be believed as Jonah.

Question 2

Table 9-1 shows the annual income of four different plumbers in Cambridgeshire across two consecutive years.

Table 9-1	Plumbers' Annual Income (in Pounds)	
Plumber	**Year 1**	**Year 2**
Drainaway	50,000	100,000
Stopdrop	60,000	70,000
Freeflow	40,000	55,000
Roundthebend	100,000	105,000
Total	250,000	330,000

Which of the following pie charts represents the percentage contribution of each plumber to the overall increase in income across all four companies?

A.

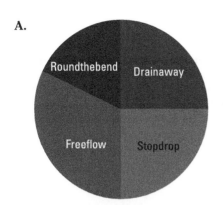

D.

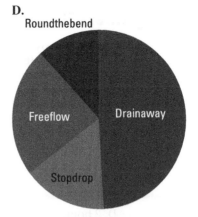

B.

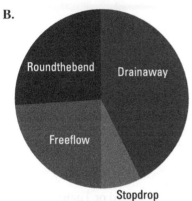

E.

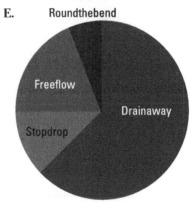

C.

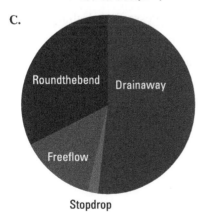

Question 3

In order to destroy a ballistic missile with its guns, a fighter jet must be level with it. An RAF jet travelling at 720 kilometres per hour (km/h) is chasing a ballistic missile travelling at 500 km/h over the Arctic Ocean. Given that they are 110 kilometres apart, how long will it take the jet to catch up with the missile?

A. 15 minutes

B. 30 minutes

C. 1 hour

D. 2 hours

E. 2 hours 20 minutes

Question 4

Oxford is west of Thame, which is west of Aylesbury. High Wycombe is east of Thame, and west of Beaconsfield. Therefore Beaconsfield must be east of:

A. Thame, but not necessarily Oxford or Aylesbury.

B. Aylesbury, but not necessarily Oxford or Thame.

C. Oxford and Thame, but not necessarily Aylesbury.

D. Oxford and Aylesbury, but not necessarily Thame.

E. Oxford, Aylesbury and High Wycombe.

Question 5

There is a concept in psychoanalysis, developed by the British analyst Donald Winnicott, called the 'good enough mother'. In brief, it suggests that a mother need not strive for eternal perfection in the care of her child, but rather that her ability to adjust appropriately as the child develops allows for yet further development. It is her inability to be perfectly empathic at all times that lets the child become a whole human being able to interact normally with others.

Indeed, within this theory, if the mother is too 'perfect' – too actively attentive, too constraining, too mindful of the child's needs and potential risks at every single moment – the child cannot learn to separate itself from the parent as it will never learn to stand on its own feet. It will never develop a healthy identity of its own.

Which one of the following can be drawn as a conclusion from the above passage?

A. A mother is 'good enough' when she is constantly aware of her child's needs.

B. If a mother is able constantly to monitor and to meet all her child's needs, the child will develop a healthy identity of its own.

C. A 'good enough' mother may not do everything perfectly all the time, but is able to respond sufficiently well that her child can develop healthily.

D. A child cannot develop unless he or she is always certain that his mother will meet his or her needs immediately.

E. Winnicott's theory of child development is widely accepted.

Scientific Knowledge and Applications Sample Questions

This section is based on the National Curriculum Key Stage 4 (essentially GCSE) standard of Biology, Chemistry, Physics and Mathematics. It frequently requires you to stretch that knowledge to arrive at the answer. In the exam, you'll have around 67 seconds per question.

Question 1

Cystic fibrosis (CF) is an autosomal recessive disorder. Jack suffers from CF and marries Sally, who doesn't suffer from the illness but is a carrier of the recessive gene. They have a daughter, Phyllis, who marries Ray. Ray's mother has CF but his father doesn't carry the recessive gene.

Given this and only this information, what are the chances that Phyllis and Ray's first child will have CF?

    A. 1 in 8

    B. 3 in 8

    C. 7 in 8

    D. The child will definitely have CF

    E. It's impossible to be sure if the child will have CF

Question 2

The concentration of a solution of Na2SO4 is 32.4 grams per litre. What is its concentration in moles per litre?

Atomic Weights: Na 23, S 32, O 16

    A. 1 mole per litre

    B. 0.5 moles per litre

    C. 0.2 moles per litre

    D. 0.1 moles per litre

    E. 0.02 moles per litre

Question 3

A car weighs 1,000 kilograms. It is raised 5 metres on a hydraulic lift over 20 seconds. Assuming perfect efficiency, how much power in watts (W) was required?

You may assume that the acceleration due to gravity is 10m/s^2.

    A. 220W

    B. 250W

    C. 500W

    D. 2,500W

    E. 100,000W

Question 4

Evaluate:

$$\sqrt{[(5 \times 10^2) + (2 \times 10^3)/(1/200) + (5 \times 10^{-3})]}$$

    A. $\sqrt{0.5}$

    B. 5

    C. 265

    D. 500

    E. 5,000

Writing Task Sample Question

A thing is not necessarily true because badly uttered, nor false because spoken magnificently.

                         — *Confessions*, St Augustine of Hippo

Discuss the above statement. What is the relationship between the way something is said and the content of the statement? What point may St Augustine be making? Should you care about how you phrase your opinions?

Checking your Answers

You can find answers and explanations to the BMAT sample questions in this section.

Aptitude and Skills

Answer 1

B and D

The possible answers are:

    A. Cassandra is less to be believed than Jonah.

    B. Jonah is not more to be believed than Cassandra.

    C. Jonah is neither more nor less to be believed as Cassandra.

    D. Cassandra is at least as much to be believed as Jonah.

You can rephrase these as algebraic expressions, where C represents Cassandra and J represents Jonah:

    A. $C < J$

    B. $J \leq C$

    C. $J = C$

    D. $C \geq J$

Mathematically, $J \leq C$ is equivalent to $C \geq J$, and so the analogous statements are B and D.

Answer 2

E.

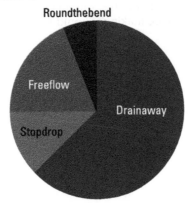

The actual increases in each plumber's income between the two years are shown in Table 9-2. They are calculated by subtracting the Year 1 income from the Year 2 income.

Table 9-2   Increases in Plumbers' Income (in Pounds)

Plumber	Year 1	Year 2	Income Increase
Drainaway	50,000	100,000	50,000
Stopdrop	60,000	70,000	10,000
Freeflow	40,000	55,000	15,000
Roundthebend	100,000	105,000	5,000
Total	250,000	330,000	80,000

Table 9-3 shows the percentages of the total income increase of $80,000 contributed by each firm.

Table 9-3   Percentage Contributions to Increase

Plumber	Percentage Contribution
Drainaway	62.50
Stopdrop	12.50
Freeflow	18.75
Roundthebend	6.25
Total	100

The only pie chart that matches this distribution is E.

You can solve this problem by doing all the above maths, but a very quick way is to notice that Drainaway contributes over half of the total increase, and the only pie charts that allocate such a large amount to its share are C and E.

You can rapidly exclude C because it gives a very large slice of the profit increase share to Roundthebend; you can see from Table 9-1 that Roundthebend's increase is proportionately small and therefore C can't be correct. E stands out as the only possible choice.

Spotting shortcuts that avoid the need to make detailed calculations is a great way to save time during the BMAT. You may find
that there are many of those.

Answer 3

B. 30 minutes

If you know the relative speed between the jet and ballistic missile,
the situation reduces to one where the jet is moving but the missile is stationary.

The relative speed is the speed of the jet minus the speed of the
ballistic missile. This is (720 − 500) = 220 km/h.

The jet is therefore moving at a relative speed of 220 km/h compared to the missile and has to cover the 110 km separating them.

Time = distance/speed = 110/220 = 0.5 hours = 30 minutes

Answer 4

C. Oxford and Thame, but not necessarily Aylesbury

You're told that Oxford is west of Thame, which is west of Aylesbury,
and that High Wycombe is east of Thame, and west of Beaconsfield.

You're asked to determine Beaconsfield's position relative to the
other locations. If Beaconsfield is east of High Wycombe and High
Wycombe is east of Thame, logically Beaconsfield must also be
east of Thame. As Thame is east of Oxford, Beaconsfield must also
be east of Oxford. However, you don't have enough information to
determine Beaconsfield's position relative to Aylesbury.

The only answer that suits is therefore C.

Answer 5

**C. A 'good enough' mother may not do everything perfectly all
the time, but is able to respond sufficiently well that her child
can develop healthily.**

You can logically conclude C from the text because the passage
states that 'a mother need not strive for eternal perfection in the
care of her child . . . it is her inability to be perfectly empathic at
all times that lets the child become a whole human being able to
interact normally with others'.

A describes a theoretically 'perfect' mother and B effectively suggests that a perfect mother is best for a child's development. Neither conclusion is supported by the passage. D is essentially a rephrased version of B. E may or may not be true, but can't be logically inferred from the information in the passage alone. Therefore C is the only correct statement, and the correct answer.

Scientific Knowledge and Applications

Answer 1
B. 3 in 8

If X is the normal gene and x the recessive gene:

> Jack is xx
>
> Sally is Xx

This means that Phyllis has a 1 in 2 chance of being xx and a 1 in 2 chance of being Xx. If she's xx, all her children will have at least one x. If she's Xx, there is a 1 in 2 chance that she'll pass on the recessive x gene. Both outcomes are equally likely and so the combined chance of her passing on a recessive x gene is:

$(1/2 \times 1) + (1/2 \times 1/2) = 1/2 + 1/4 = 3/4$

Ray's mother is xx but his father is XX. Ray must therefore be Xx, and the chance of him passing on an x gene to his children 1 in 2. Combining this 1 in 2 chance with Sally's 3 in 4 chance yields 3 in 8.

$1/2 \times 3/4 = 3/8$ or 3 in 8

Answer 2
C. 0.2 moles per litre

You're asked to calculate the concentration of the solution in moles per litre from the concentration in grams per litre.

Moles = mass/molecular weight = $32.4/[(23 \times 2) + 32 + (16 \times 4)]$ = $32.4/162 = 0.2$ moles

Therefore the concentration is 0.2 moles per litre.

Answer 3

D. 2,500W

The watt is a unit of power. You're asked to determine the power required to lift the car:

Power = work done/time taken

Work done = force applied × distance travelled

Force = mass × acceleration

Combining the above:

Power = (mass × acceleration × distance travelled)/time taken = $(1000 \times 10 \times 5)/20 = 2500W$

Answer 4

D. 500

$\sqrt{[(5 \times 10^2) + (2 \times 10^3)/(1/200) + (5 \times 10^{-3})]}$

$= \sqrt{[(500 + 2000)/(0.005 + 0.005)]}$

$= \sqrt{(2500/0.01)} = \sqrt{250000} = 500$

 This calculation is relatively simple, but with such a large number of brackets to process correctly, and with a range of different powers and signs, you can easily make careless errors. Take the calculation one step at a time.

Writing Task

A thing is not necessarily true because badly uttered, nor false because spoken magnificently.

— *Confessions*, St Augustine of Hippo

Model answer

St Augustine of Hippo, patron saint of such diverse groups as brewers and theologians, is renowned as one of the greatest Christian thinkers of all time. His statement that 'A thing is not necessarily true because badly uttered, nor false because spoken magnificently' is a bold challenge to two commonplace, but opposing, worldviews.

The first worldview is one of rigorous logic: facts are all that matter and if the facts of an argument are correct, then everything else is irrelevant. The second, opposing worldview is that facts are irrelevant because people are more amenable to a good story than to cold argument or painful truth. What you can persuade someone to believe is all that matters.

Augustine's quote illustrates that both approaches are false. He separates reality from presentation but does not deny the importance of either. To Augustine, truth is absolute; something is either correct or it is false. For him, it is illogical to suggest that something must be true because it is presented beautifully and equally illogical to suggest it must be true because it is presented more humbly. The style of presentation and the nature of reality are not different sides of the same coin, but entirely separate attributes.

However, implicit in Augustine's statement is a recognition that humans are not pure thinking machines; we are influenced by beauty and passion. An elegant argument can be used to persuade, regardless of truth. Although the saintly may always be able to distinguish what merely glitters and what is gold, the rest of us can be less discerning.

Until everyone is intelligent and insightful enough to separate consistently the truth of an argument from its persuasive power, how we present our opinion still matters. But Augustine's quote reminds us to retain a deeper awareness of what is truth, even while constructing an argument that meets our needs.

It is a practical philosophy of personal integrity and good insight, and acknowledgement of the seductive power of persuasion.

Explanation

The answer is 328 words long. With neat handwriting this fits onto the single side of lined A4 paper provided for the Writing Task in the BMAT. The essay is fluent, well written and legible, with no spelling, grammatical or punctuation errors. As a result, it scores very highly on the A to E Quality of English component of the marking scheme.

The answer begins with a short introduction and proceeds to address each element of the question in turn. It introduces Augustine's statement, considers the point he may have been making, and assesses its relevance to our times. The candidate acknowledges the power of the statement but doesn't blindly accept it, pointing out that not everyone is capable of meeting the high intellectual standards it demands.

The candidate then provides a nuanced judgement in her conclusion: she takes on board the essential veracity of the argument but tempers that with an acceptance of the practical reality of the world.

A thoughtful and balanced discussion like this would score very well on the Quality of Content component of the marking scheme. It answers all aspects of the question, makes excellent use of the material, and generates a strong counter-proposition. The ideas are expressed logically and the conclusion is succinct and compelling.

Chapter 10

Getting to Grips with the GAMSAT

In This Chapter
▶ Introducing the GAMSAT
▶ Applying for and sitting the test
▶ Familiarising yourself with the test's structure

A few universities require graduate applicants to sit the Graduate Australian Medical School Admissions Test (GAMSAT) as part of their selection procedure. For this reason, we discuss the nature of this test, tell you which UK institutions use it, and show you how to prepare for it.

Introducing the GAMSAT

The GAMSAT was developed in 1995 by a group of medical schools in Australia to help them select medical students. The test was brought to the UK around the turn of the century and is now used by a small handful of British medical schools.

The GAMSAT tests your reasoning ability rather than being a test of pure knowledge. It consists of multiple choice questions on verbal reasoning and scientific topics plus an essay section. It's designed to test whether students have the skills and knowledge to cope with the challenges of a medical degree.

Taking the GAMSAT

Table 10-1 lists the medical courses and universities that require the GAMSAT as part of their selection process.

Table 10-1	Universities and Courses Requiring the GAMSAT
University	*UCAS Course Code and Course*
Nottingham	A101 (Medicine: graduate entry 4-year programme)
Peninsula College of Medicine and Dentistry	A100 (Medicine: non-direct school leavers only)
St George's, University of London	A101 (Medicine: graduate entry 4-year programme)
Swansea	A101 (Medicine: graduate entry 4-year programme)

Getting the dates right

The exact dates for the GAMSAT cycle (registration, testing, and publication of results) vary annually, though usually by no more than a few days. GAMSAT maintains its own website with the relevant dates. The UK website is http://gamsat.acer.edu.au/gamsat-uk and the parent site has information on test dates in other countries too.

GAMSAT scores are equivalent whether you sit the exam in Australia, Ireland or the UK. You can use your score for a period of two years before needing to sit the exam again. There's no limit to the number of times you may sit the test. If you have multiple scores, your highest aggregate score can be used to support your medical school application. This isn't done automatically, however, unless you link the GAMSAT accounts. To take advantage of this system you need to register your scores with UCAS by following the relevant instructions within the Results section of your GAMSAT UK account (check out the later section 'Registering for the GAMSAT').

As an example of the approximate dates to keep in mind, Table 10-2 lists the dates for a typical cycle in the UK.

Table 10-2	Key GAMSAT UK Dates
Event	*Date*
Registration opens	4 June
Standard entry closing date	10 August
Last date for entry (late fees apply)	20 August
Last date for refund of fees for cancellation (administrative charge applies)	20 August
Test date	21 September
Results day	Typically 6–8 weeks after the test date

You don't have a choice about the GAMSAT test date. Plan ahead and make sure that you don't have any other major appointments or commitments in the week preceding the exam.

If your medical school choices mean that you also need to sit the UKCAT (Chapters 6 and 7) or the BMAT (Chapters 8 and 9), we suggest that you try to space out these tests. Some people do argue that revising for one test helps with the others, but, on balance, we feel that having some downtime between tests makes the overall process easier.

If you need to cancel your test, you can get a refund provided you cancel before the deadline (indicated in Table 10-2).

Registering for the GAMSAT

To register for the GAMSAT, open an account at the website (http://gamsat.acer.edu.au/gamsat-uk).

The entry fee is £222 provided that you register for the test before the standard entry closing date (see Table 10-2). After that, you can still register as long as you submit before the last date for entry and pay £60 in late fees.

UK test centres are located in Bristol, London, Nottingham, Sheffield and Swansea. You can choose a preferred centre when you register but aren't guaranteed the centre of your choice.

Candidates with a disability that may impair their test performance should submit a statement to this effect by the standard closing date, together with supporting evidence.

Preparing for test day

The GAMSAT organisers email your admission ticket to you approximately two weeks before the test date, along with information on the precise time and location of the test.

Make sure that you know where you're going on test day and arrive early to allow for any administrative formalities. Bring a pencil, an eraser and a black or blue pen. You aren't permitted to take anything else into the test room itself.

You aren't permitted to use a calculator.

Bring your admission ticket with you, along with a valid passport, photo driving licence or certified letter of identification with a passport photo stamped by the certifier.

Performing well on test day

The GAMSAT is a long, challenging exam. You may find these tips helpful to remain focused on test day:

- ✔ Arrive early so you're ready to start on time.
- ✔ Read all questions quickly but carefully.
- ✔ Avoid skim-reading, especially on multiple choice sections.
- ✔ Don't be intimidated by unfamiliar topics; examiners are looking for logical thought, not encyclopaedic knowledge.
- ✔ Write so that examiners can comfortably read your handwriting (if your writing is near illegible, avoid using cursive script).
- ✔ Don't spend too much time on questions you can't answer; move on to the next question and keep your cool.
- ✔ Accept that the GAMSAT's a tough exam; just focus on doing your best.

Deconstructing the GAMSAT

The GAMSAT is a pen, pencil and paper exam that lasts a whopping 5 hours 30 minutes, with a one-hour lunch break between Sections II and III. The test consists of three sections, each timed separately (as we describe in the later section 'Considering the time pressures'):

- ✔ **Section I – Reasoning in Humanities and Social Sciences:** Contains multiple choice questions.

- ✔ **Section II – Written Communication:** Contains two essay questions.

- ✔ **Section III – Reasoning in Biological and Physical Sciences:** Contains multiple choice questions.

Examining the sections

We now go through each of these sections in detail, so you know how best to prepare.

Reasoning in Humanities and Social Sciences

This section tests generic skills often used in undergraduate study, including understanding written or pictorial information, constructing logical arguments and problem solving. It tests whether you can interpret information to draw accurate and appropriate conclusions.

Many of the techniques we suggest in Chapter 6 for preparing for the Verbal Reasoning subtest of the UKCAT exam also apply to preparing for this section of the GAMSAT.

Written Communication

This section usually offers five or six propositions, of which you need to choose and discuss two. The propositions can be on any topic and typically at least one has a socio-cultural aspect. As with the BMAT essay, the Written Communication section tests your ability to reason around a topic and express your thoughts cogently.

You can't possibly research every topic that may come up in this section. The GAMSAT doesn't expect you to be familiar with the subjects of its propositions but to be able to use logical principles and general knowledge to discuss them.

If the question is about an ethical dilemma, remember that it can usually be explored by thinking sequentially about its impact on various domains such as health, education, civil rights, state needs, societal benefit and environmental impact among many others. After you've explored these domains, weigh them up to reach a balanced conclusion.

Practise writing timed essays around different topics, because doing so gets you into the habit of exploring a topic quickly from many angles.

The Written Communication section also assesses the quality of your English: revise the basic elements of grammar, style and punctuation. *The Economist* (at www.economist.com/styleguide/ introduction) and the BBC (www.bbc.co.uk/journalism/ skills/writing) offer good style guides on their websites.

Reasoning in Biological and Physical Sciences

As in Section I, the questions are presented in a multiple-choice format. You need to be familiar with Biology and Chemistry up to about first-year undergraduate level and Physics up to about A-level.

If you haven't recently studied any of the sciences, we suggest revising them up to at least A-level standard.

Considering the time pressures

Students consistently report that the time pressure in the GAMSAT is intense, especially in Section III. Table 10-3 indicates the time allowed for each section and the number of questions per section together with the time per question.

Table 10-3	Timing for the GAMSAT Sections		
Section	**Time Allowed**	**Questions**	**Time per Question**
Reasoning in Humanities and Social Sciences	100 minutes	75 items	80 seconds
Written Communication	60 minutes	2 items	30 minutes
Reasoning in Biological and Physical Sciences	170 minutes	110 items	Roughly 93 seconds

The times per item give you a general idea of how to pace yourself in each section. Naturally, some questions are harder than others, and you may find yourself spending a little longer on the harder ones. This means that you need to be brisker on the simpler ones.

Practice questions are available at `http://gamsat.acer.edu.au/prepare/preparation-materials`. Working with practice questions is immensely helpful and we strongly recommend that you do that.

Making out the marking

Sections I and III of the GAMSAT are marked based on the number of correct responses you give on the test. The test doesn't use *negative marking,* which means that your score doesn't go down if you give a wrong answer; you just fail to gain marks on that question.

If you don't know the answer, guess! You can't actively lose marks.

Your marks for Sections I and III are each scaled and calibrated to give a score out of 100. These scores aren't straightforward percentages, and also take into account how other candidates perform.

Section II (Writing Communication) is also marked out of 100 but is graded by human beings rather than by computer. Marks are awarded for both the quality of the content and the quality of your English. As you might expect, a reasoned, supported and structured line of argument attracts the highest marks.

Studying the scores

As well as section scores, you're issued an overall GAMSAT score. This score out of 100 is based on a weighted formula that combines the individual section scores:

Overall Score = (1 × Section I + 1 × Section II + 2 × Section III) ÷ 4

This equation accords a lot of weight to the science section, but you do need to score reasonably well in the other sections too.

Universities don't consistently reveal details of how they use the GAMSAT to select medical students and the selection criteria can vary between years. However, they generally want to see a good overall score with a more or less uniform distribution between the three sections. In previous years, scores of around 50–55 have met minimum requirements; in more recent years, intensifying competition has called for scores of a little over 60.

If you don't perform well in the GAMSAT, try to put the result out of your mind. Focus on doing well in what still remains in your control.

Part III
Preparing for Interviews

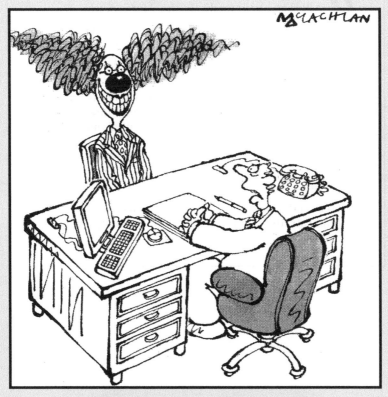

'Ok, I'll take your word for it that you're happy with who you are.'

In this part...

Part III is all about medical school interviews.

The vast majority of medical schools interview prospective students. For many applicants this will be the first time they attend a formal interview and it can be a nerve-wracking experience.

Preparation is the key to confidence and success. In this part we begin by reviewing the various interview formats and then cover in detail most of the potential questions that you'll face. We also explore some frequently asked medical and ethical issues. Candidates who can discuss these issues maturely and thoughtfully will be ahead of their competitors.

This part ends with a review of your options after interview, including strategies on choosing between competing offers.

Chapter 11

Performing Well in Interviews

. . . .

In This Chapter

▶ Understanding how medical school interviews work

▶ Investigating what interviewers want to know

▶ Preparing effectively for interviews

▶ Considering how you come across

. . . .

*I*nterviews are a vital part of the selection process at most medical schools, though not all. Southampton and Edinburgh don't interview undergraduates, although Edinburgh does interview graduate applicants.

We don't recommend applying to a medical school solely because it doesn't interview. Job interviews are a part of life and with practice and preparation you've nothing to fear. In fact, they're an opportunity for you to prove that you're a great candidate and will fit in well.

In this chapter we explain what medical school interviews are like, how to prepare for them and what interviewers are looking for. Our discussion may also help you with interviews later in life and hopefully give you a better insight into effective interpersonal interaction.

Knowing What to Expect

In this section we dispel the fear of medical school interviews by laying bare the shortlisting process and dissecting the interview format.

Getting shortlisted

Medical schools interview a relatively small proportion of all its applicants. As a result, they need to use a shortlisting approach to narrow the field of applicants.

The formula that medical schools use to shortlist candidates for interview isn't uniform or straightforward. Some institutions apply a weighted formula based on your existing and predicted grades, and a scoring of your personal statement and selection test results. Others are more qualitative or subjective in their approach. Few medical schools explicitly describe their criteria.

In general, you don't need to worry about the shortlisting formula because it isn't going to alter your approach to applying. There are, however, two exceptions to this advice:

- ✔ Universities that require the BMAT (which we describe in Chapter 8) consider it a vital part of the shortlisting process. Therefore, don't apply to BMAT universities if you won't do well in the exam.

- ✔ Some UKCAT universities place inordinate weight on a strong exam result; if you sit the UKCAT early and do poorly, avoid applying to medical schools that weigh it strongly (see Chapter 6 for details of the UKCAT). Historically, these UKCAT-heavy universities are Barts and The London, Durham, Glasgow, Hull/York, Queen's University Belfast, Sheffield and Warwick. The other UKCAT universities use the scores as a smaller part of their formula or in borderline cases only. Note that there is a trend away from using the UKCAT score as a crude cut-off for shortlisting. For instance, in 2011 Sheffield applied a rigid cut-off of 2870 but in 2012 they only used the UKCAT as a component of their overall shortlisting process.

If you follow the advice that we provide in Parts I and II, you have every chance of doing well enough to be considered for interview.

Knowing the interview format

The format of medical school interview varies widely from one institution to another. A clear majority follow the traditional model of one or two 15–20-minute interviews. The interview panel ranges from two to four people drawn from a pool of experienced selectors, sometimes together with a final-year medical student.

Interviews are frequently *semi-structured* which means that the panel has a range of pre-planned topics to ask about, with certain pre-determined replies gaining the highest marks. But the interview is also flexible, and interviewers can ask new questions and move onto related topics if that's the best way of assessing the interviewee. Manchester and Warwick go further and have additional group sessions in an attempt to specifically test team-working and communication skills.

A few medical schools feel that the semi-structured interview approach is unfair because it benefits those with good social skills. As most people expect a doctor to have these skills, selecting partly on this basis seems fair to us, but a minority of schools use more structured interview methods instead.

The following universities use a Multiple Mini Interview (MMI) or similar Objective Structured Clinical Exam (OSCE) approach for their medical school interviews:

- ✔ Aberdeen
- ✔ Dundee
- ✔ Edinburgh (graduates only)
- ✔ King's College London (graduates only)
- ✔ Queen's University Belfast
- ✔ St George's
- ✔ University of East Anglia
- ✔ University of Leicester

At the time of writing, Glasgow uses an MMI format for dentistry but not for medicine, whereas Aberdeen has now adopted the MMI style for both dentistry and medicine. We suspect that Glasgow is likely to follow suit.

Multiple Mini Interviews consist of a series of different tasks, each assessed by a different set of examiners. You move from one station to another at regular intervals, usually prompted by a bell ringing. The number of stations and time spent at each varies among medical schools, but eight stations of five minutes each with one minute between stations is typical.

A station may take the form of a discussion with the examiner, a piece of written or pictorial information to interpret, or even a role-play. Each mini interview tests a different skill, for example, academic ability, empathy, team working and decision-making.

In our opinion the topics tested in MMIs are very similar to those evaluated in traditional semi-structured interviews, but the latter seems to be a less artificial interaction. It mimics the real nature of a doctor–patient consultation more closely than the rigid MMI format, which is more anxiety-provoking as a result of the bell ringing and having to move from one station to the next.

If you think that you'll perform better at MMIs (and they certainly have their advocates), by all means apply to the medical schools that practise it.

The topics and skills tested in an MMI setting are substantially similar to those tested in a semi-structured interview. For that reason, we focus in this chapter on the types of questions asked rather than on the specific types of interviews.

Putting Yourself in the Interviewers' Shoes

In this section we help you answer the question: 'What do medical school interviewers want to know?' They already have plenty of evidence about your academic achievements, so the bulk of the interview is likely to focus on other areas.

Interviewers want to test your commitment to medicine and knowledge of medical practice, your ability to think quickly and make decisions, and how well you communicate and empathise with others. They're also looking for a sense of curiosity about the world, a willingness to learn and show initiative, and good ethical awareness. To search for these traits, they explore your decision to become a doctor and apply to their medical school, and test your soft skills by confronting you with difficult or controversial hypothetical, current and historical scenarios.

When an interviewer asks you a question, don't just consider its superficial meaning. Work out why you're being asked that question and tailor your answer to that purpose.

For example, if an interviewer asks about your work experience, they don't want to hear a long list of hospitals you've worked in. They want to hear what *kinds* of work experience you did and what you took away from these experiences. Did they teach you something new? Did they change your preconceptions about medicine? How did they motivate you to apply to medical school?

Always be on the lookout for this type of unspoken hidden question and address it overtly. Do not rehearse fully-scripted answers: they frequently sound false and wooden when delivered in interviews, and run the risk of not precisely answering the question. Using a mental bullet-point approach is far better. Hold the main points you want to discuss in the back of your mind and wheel them out whenever an opportunity arises. As a result, you sound more natural and convincing and also maintain a good sense of awareness about the conversation you're having. This knowledge lets you judge how the interview is going and adapt accordingly. For example, if the interviewers seem encouraging and interested in what you're saying, you can expand on your discussion points. If they're clearly itching to move on to another topic, you can opt to quickly summarise your points.

Interviews are a subjective process, no matter how much the interviewers may be trying to be structured and objective. Good interpersonal skills aid good communication and make a difference to the impression you make.

Getting Ready for Interviews

Medical school interviews are pretty short. But the build-up is much longer and there's much you can do to ensure that you create a good impression on the day.

Arriving on time

This advice sounds simple but you'd be surprised how many candidates turn up late for interviews or arrive flustered and uncomfortable. Here's a straightforward checklist for arriving on time:

- ✔ **Read the information the medical school sends you in advance.** This usually contains the time of your interview, the time at which you're expected to arrive at the interview centre, a list of the paperwork required (such as a photo ID) and maybe even a map of the area. Pay close attention to instructions about dress code (check out the later section 'Looking the part' as well), arrival times and administrative formalities.

- ✔ **Don't assume that you'll have a trouble-free journey, especially if travelling to London or far from home.** Leave early, plan your route carefully, make sure that you have a fully charged mobile phone and have a range of payment options in case of emergencies. But remember to turn your phone off when you reach your destination, as the ironic comedy value of your *Casualty* theme ringtone is very unlikely to raise a laugh from your interviewers!

✔ **Obtain a paper map of the area.** People often use sat-nav and mobiles to get to unfamiliar destinations, which is great until they suddenly stop functioning. Feel free to use them but do keep a paper back-up . . . just in case.

✔ **Aim to arrive early.** Doing so gives you leeway in case of traffic jams or last-minute crises. If you hate hanging around places ahead of time (and frankly, interview waiting rooms aren't the most pleasant of environments), you can always find a local cafe to kill some time in. The point is to be in the local area early.

Going in with the right attitude

Interviewers want to see rounded human beings with a positive but realistic outlook on life, and people who are enthusiastic and knowledgeable about a career in medicine. Therefore, you want to appear polite, professional and respectful. Arrogance, rudeness, or snobbery almost always results in rejection.

The problem is that selection interviews are stressful and when people are stressed, they can behave in ways they normally wouldn't. Well-hidden personality quirks can surface and suddenly you say something glib or flippant that makes you sound potentially unsafe as a doctor.

Managing your nerves so that you retain enough tension to be alert and quick-witted without panicking and saying something silly is a difficult skill (we provide a few tips on at least *looking* relaxed in the later section 'Sitting comfortably'). Practice does make a huge difference, so in the run-up to your interview find colleagues or an enthusiastic teacher or careers adviser with whom to bounce off questions and answers.

If you know someone who regularly carries out job interviews, ask them to role-play with you. Or attend a course on interview technique that features mock-interview practice sessions.

The point of practice is to discover how to stay relaxed under pressure and maintain your composure. As a result you project the aura of a competent, modest, thoughtful, caring and decisive professional.

We provide more guidance on specific questions and topics in Chapters 12 and 13, but here's some general advice when you're discussing topics with interviewers:

- **Don't be over-inclusive:** Waffling and tangential answers distract interviewers and leave you less time to score strongly.

- **Substantiate and personalise:** For example, if asked about your extracurricular activities, don't just list them but try to explain why you chose them and what you learned from them.

- **Express your strengths objectively:** Let the facts speak for themselves by explaining how you succeeded at difficult tasks. For instance, if questioned about your organisational skills, give an example of a time when you put them to good use.

- **Avoid highlighting negative aspects:** This sounds obvious, but people tend to make self-deprecatory jokes when under pressure. Remember to focus on your strengths. Knowing your weaknesses is important, but keep them in context instead of just throwing them into the conversation.

- **Bear in mind that interviewers are trying to offer you a place, not to catch you out:** This is a cliché but true; they really do want to see you at your best. Walk into an interview aiming to shine, not just to minimise damage.

- **Show your ability to understand issues:** Give both sides of complicated ethical dilemmas, volunteering your opinion only at the end of that discussion.

- **Remember that in many cases, especially with regard to medical or political dilemmas, there are no right or easy answers:** Be open and honest about difficulty, uncertainty and risk. If you don't know an answer, say so, and then describe how you'd find the answer. This may not sound ideal, but it's much better than digging yourself into a hole or, worse still, appearing dishonest.

Knowing your brief

You have to be consistent with your UCAS application and echo what is already on your personal statement (this is another reason to give a lot of consideration to your personal statement). If you change your story now, you come across as flighty or dishonest.

Before your interview, look back at what you wrote in your statement. Print off a copy and keep it in your pocket on the day so
that you can remind yourself of its contents before going into the
interview room. Also, review the specific medical school you're
interviewing at. Re-read its website and prospectus and try to get a
feel for what it's like and what sort of candidates it's looking for.

This preparation helps you to tailor your answers to the interviewers and avoid asking about a topic that you should be familiar
with or saying something that might immediately disqualify you.
For example, you don't want to say to interviewers at Hull York
Medical School that you really hate the Problem Based Learning
approach!

Controlling the Signals You Send Out

Communication experts suggest that good impressions aren't just
a matter of what you say but also how you say it. Appearance,
body language and tone of voice are critical components of good
communication skills. You may think that placing importance
on such matters is unfair, but their relevance is a fact of life.
Psychological studies suggest that when forming opinions about
others, people are greatly influenced by first and last impressions
(*primacy* and *recency* effects) and less by the intermediate content.
Have a look at *Body Language For Dummies* by Elizabeth Kuhnke
(Wiley) to discover how to let your voice and body do the talking.

During an interview your aim is to maximise the impact that you
are making. How you look and speak need to be congruent with
what you say, and the whole package needs to work together to
reinforce the message that you'll be a great doctor.

Put yourself in the shoes of patients talking to their doctor: they
need to have confidence in that person. Good communication
skills immediately project that trustworthiness and are a part of
the therapeutic alliance between doctors and their patients.

Although a polished appearance and masterful voice control are
never going to be enough to get you into medical school on their
own, looking and sounding professional does eliminate unnecessary distractions from your interview answers. If a medical school
is going to turn you down, let it be because it doesn't think you're
a strong enough candidate and not because you distract an interviewer with your overpowering aftershave!

Looking the part

We divide appearance into how you look and how you physically behave during the interview.

Dressing smartly

Some interviews specify a dress code. If they do, follow it scrupulously. If they insist on casual clothes, pick items within that category that are clean, ironed, fit and appear conservative.

If they don't specify casual or business dress, err on the smarter end of the spectrum. Make sure that everything fits well. If this interview is your first time in a suit, wear it a few times ahead of the interview so that you feel comfortable in it. The same advice applies if you buy a new pair of shoes; you don't want painful blisters on interview day!

If you're not sure what business clothes are appropriate for interviews, here are some suggestions for men:

- ✔ **A conservative suit in navy or charcoal grey:** A two- or three-button single-breasted front is always classic, though a double-breasted suit isn't the end of the world. If you don't have a suit, an odd jacket such as a navy blazer, paired with smart grey trousers, is acceptable.

- ✔ **A white shirt in plain fabric, preferably with a moderately spread collar and button cuffs:** If your shirt needs cufflinks, pick discreet ones in a silver or gold colour. Alternatively, a similarly styled pale-blue shirt is fine.

- ✔ **Black shoes:** They should be clean and reasonably polished. Laced oxfords are a classic choice.

- ✔ **A tie in a colour that complements your suit without being too bright, such as navy or dark burgundy:** Choose a solid textured tie such as a grenadine weave or a conservative pindot or stripe pattern.

- ✔ **No pocket handkerchiefs:** Also, steer clear of strong or excessive cologne, earrings, piercings and other distracting details.

In addition, ensure that you're clean-shaven or have neatly-groomed facial hair and that your fingernails are trim and clean.

Dressing for the part (or not!)

One of us recalls wearing a very 1980s double-breasted suit with a navy polka dot tie to a medical school interview and still getting in, only to push the boat further years later in an equally successful job interview, wearing a tie with a floral pattern better suited to wallpaper and an overly flouncy silk pocket handkerchief.

So although conservative clothes are a good idea, don't feel too constrained by our advice!

For women, we suggest:

- ✔ **A conservative business suit, with skirt or trousers, and a shirt or blouse that's not too revealing:** If you opt for a skirt, avoid going higher than just above the knee.

- ✔ **Court shoes with a modest heel:** Or flats if you dislike heels.

- ✔ **Hosiery at your discretion:** But avoid garish colours.

- ✔ **You can be a little braver with colour and pattern than men if you want:** But a conservative look is still the most appropriate option for a serious interview.

- ✔ **Hair under control, whether worn up or down:** Also, apply make-up with a light and careful touch.

- ✔ **Earrings are fine:** But keep them small and discreet rather than large and jangling.

- ✔ **Strong perfumes should be avoided:** They can be distracting and some people are genuinely allergic to them.

These lists are simply guidance for a conservative, interview-appropriate look that doesn't offer any hostages to fortune. They're not meant to be exhaustive or prescriptive. In any case, a somewhat eccentric appearance can definitely be compensated for by a substantive interview performance (as the nearby 'Dressing for the part (or not!)' sidebar confirms).

Sitting comfortably

Think about how the people you know look when sitting down: some slouch, others sit upright; some constantly fidget, others rarely move.

In an interview, you want to appear interested and relaxed even though you may be feeling a mix of frustration and anxiety. Aim to be like the proverbial swan, gliding gracefully across the surface of the lake while paddling furiously under the water.

Tips that help you look poised even under stress include:

- **Maintaining an *open body posture*:** This means avoiding crossing your arms and appearing defensive and surly. Crossing your legs isn't the end of civilisation, but the best approach is to sit comfortably with legs uncrossed and together.

- **Keeping your hands still:** Use gestures to emphasise important points instead of gesticulating wildly.

- **Sitting up, leaning forward slightly:** Don't slouch and don't lean so far forward so that you look anxious or desperate.

- **Maintaining good eye contact:** Especially with the person who asked you the last question.

You can take eye contact too far; you don't want to be the candidate who fixes the interviewer with an unwavering stare! Natural eye contact comes and goes but on balance is maintained more often than not.

If you're not sure how you look when asked questions, try videoing yourself. You'll probably hate the results the first time, but it's a useful way to notice and remove distracting habits.

Controlling body language becomes easier the more you practise it. Looking confident is an art and helps you engage positively with other people. Doctors need to inspire confidence and consciously working on this skill pays dividends.

Sounding the part

As well as appearance and body language (which we describe in the preceding section), how you speak is also an important element of communication. The aim isn't to recreate a standardised received-pronunciation accent if you don't have one, but to use clear diction and a controlled tone. People tend to speak faster and louder when feeling excited, mangle sentences when anxious and mumble when feeling low. Without care, your voice can betray your inner thoughts and feelings.

As with body language, you can control your tone of voice with practice. Aim to sound calm and positive, without being loud or rapid. Let yourself speak a little faster when discussing topics you're enthusiastic about, and slow down slightly when wishing to demonstrate thoughtfulness.

Chapter 12

Preparing for Common Interview Questions

. . . .

In This Chapter

▶ Dealing with questions about yourself

▶ Demonstrating your interest in medicine

▶ Getting hypothetical

▶ Interviewing the interviewers

. . . .

*I*nterviewers tend to ask candidates similar questions and so many of those you face in a typical medical school interview are predictable. The others are likely to be on such varied topics that preparing for them is either impossible or inefficient.

Medical school interviews are part of a competitive selection process, which means that if you answer the predictable questions very well you're already ahead of competitors who don't. Then you only need to do moderately well on the more unpredictable questions and you're well on your way into medical school.

 The best answers to interview questions are ones that are honest and personal, but integrated within a structure that makes practical sense to the interviewer. Our aim in this chapter is to help you discover how to contextualise your individuality in this way, because that's the mark of a good interviewee.

We cover the questions comprising the predictable parts of the interview concerning your personal life, career intentions and hypothetical scenarios. We discuss structuring your answers so that they are comprehensive without sounding rehearsed. We also provide some hints on how to approach the more unusual questions.

We include sample answers only to highlight how to apply the skills we describe in practice. Don't memorise these samples – that would be one of the worst ways to prepare. Sample answers by definition can't reflect your own circumstances and so if you memorise them, you're sure to sound scripted and false and are likely to be rejected. (Plus if everyone uses the same answer, interviewers might well smell a rat!)

Talking about Yourself

After the initial pleasantries, interviewers frequently start by asking you a series of questions to probe your motives for applying and your personal history.

Taking control of the interview: 'Tell me about yourself'

This open-ended question often unnerves students, especially applicants to undergraduate courses with less life (and interview) experience. Like most questions, it can crop up in different guises, from the less intimidating 'Talk me through your personal statement' to the more challenging 'Why are you here today?' and even the rather frightening 'Why should we select you over the other candidates waiting outside?'.

Instead of seeing it as scary, view this question as an opportunity to frame the information about yourself in a positive manner. Think about what the interviewers are trying to find out. They don't want your unedited life history, full of trivial details such as where you were born and what nursery school you went to. Instead, they want to hear a coherent explanation for applying to medical school that's rooted in an ethical and responsible approach to life. They also need to know that you're capable of completing the course and coping with life as a doctor.

Armed with this knowledge, you can see that what they really want to elicit is much the same information as on your UCAS personal statement (which we help you to write in Chapter 5). What you say in the interview needs to echo what you originally wrote, or else you risk coming across as flighty or dishonest.

Structure your answer in the same logical way as you did your personal statement. Begin by summarising your motivation for studying medicine and then reinforce this with some information about your academic record, work experience and non-academic skills.

Don't just list information, however, because this quickly becomes dry and artificial. Instead, use anecdotes and examples to demonstrate the truth of your statements.

In the following example, notice how the candidate's answer exploits the initial vague and open-ended nature of the question. It wrests some control of the interview away from the interviewer and towards the candidate, allowing the person to discuss a topic he knows very well – himself:

> *I'm here because I want to study medicine at this university.*
>
> *I've got a strong academic record, spanning the sciences and humanities, and I love working with people. I want to be in a profession where it's possible to express my interest in science and in people. Medicine is almost unique in that respect, and I also like the fact that I'll be using those skills to make a positive difference to people's lives.*

At this point, as you pause, you may get interrupted and asked a follow-up question. If not, expand on your opening statement of intent:

> *It was a big decision. I'm working hard to meet my teachers' predictions of 2 A*s and 2 As at A-level, but I also had to prove to myself that I'm suited to life as a doctor.*
>
> *I did a range of work experience at a general hospital and with my GP. I shadowed doctors at the hospital in their clinics and on the wards, and helped out in the pharmacy and reception at the GP practice. I also do regular voluntary work at a local hospice.*
>
> *It's remarkable just how broad medical life is. All these different branches are working towards the same aim – helping sick people and their families through exceptionally tough times – but the settings are very different from each other. The pressures are also very different.*
>
> *In the hospital, doctors constantly deal with a large, changing population of very unwell people. It's a real challenge to manage that workload, triaging different patients' needs correctly. In the GP surgery you get to know people better over time but because there are so many people with relatively minor problems, it can sometimes be harder to spot something serious presenting with low-level symptoms.*
>
> *What's common to both settings is the administrative and management burden; all the doctors I saw spent a lot of time ensuring that they were up to date on that aspect of their work, despite the occasional grumble about it!*

Hospice work is quite different. It's slower-paced and staff, myself included, have more time to talk to patients. That has the flipside of feeling it more when they pass away. Everyone supports each other and there are sessions for staff to talk about how they're feeling, which helps.

My hobbies also help me to de-stress. I'm pretty active in the school's hockey team. Only the second team, admittedly, but I'm captain this year, which is great fun. I have to think more about the team as a unit and how to bring the best out of everyone and our results this year are improving.

On balance, I'm a positive, thoughtful and hard-working person. From what I've seen, those are traits that should help me as a doctor. Medicine isn't something I've decided to do on a whim; I've thought about it carefully. I'd love to have the opportunity to study it here.

The applicant uses the opportunity to talk about his academic record, rooting it in fact (predicted grades). He then covers his motivation to study medicine, showing insight into his personality and demonstrating practical experience in a range of settings. He talks about the downsides of medicine, as well as the good parts, and is down-to-earth and realistic. The discussion of his hobbies shows a good mix of humility and leadership. Finally, he rounds off the answer with a concise summary of his reasons for applying.

This answer may seem a bit long, but when said out loud it takes only a minute or two, making it a realistic length.

Don't be frightened by open-ended questions. Vague questions are a boon because they offer the opportunity for personal expression and for taking some control over the course of the interview. In fact, the questions with only one possible correct short answer are trickier because they often test your factual knowledge, and if you simply don't know the answer you have little opportunity to talk around the subject! For example, some medical schools that require Biology A-level may decide to ask you a specific question that you should be able to answer from your knowledge of the A-level syllabus.

Showing your motivation: 'Why do you want to study medicine?'

Interviewers generally ask this question to ensure that your desire to study medicine stems from an appropriate and realistic understanding of the profession (and not that you once saw an old episode of *ER* and decided that George Clooney makes for an excellent role model!).

Concentrate on demonstrating a clear and ethical motivation. The best answers are honest and straightforward explanations of your motives and tend to fall into two broad categories:

- ✔ **Life story:** This discusses a key event or series of events in your life that brought you into contact with the medical world. You can use it to discuss what inspired you about medicine, and why the life of a doctor appeals to you so much. You can then ground your answer in practical matters by discussing your work experience.

- ✔ **Personal insight:** This requires a clear explanation of your strengths and weaknesses, allied to recognition that the role of a doctor matches that profile well. Broaden this answer with a statement about the enjoyment and fulfilment you hope to get out of being a doctor.

Both strategies hit the same basic 'notes' but approach the answer from opposite ends of the spectrum. The story angle starts off with inspiration and ends with practicalities; the insight approach starts off with the practicalities and ends with inspiration.

 Choose the style that best reflects your own personality and reasons for applying to study medicine. Whatever approach you use, weave in a strand referencing your communication skills, because medical schools value this trait highly.

Here's a sample answer for the personal insight approach:

> *I really enjoy talking to people. I find it fascinating trying to understand what makes them tick and figuring out how to help them and solve problems. I want to work in a job where I get to do this in a meaningful way. I've always done very well at school, particularly enjoying biology and chemistry, so when thinking about careers and the fact I like working with people and solving problems, the idea of studying medicine quickly moved to the forefront of my mind.*

> *At first, I didn't know much about being a doctor, so I had to do a lot of research. That included talking to doctors and medical students, and doing work experience at my local general hospital.*

> *I found out that the job can be really tough at times. There's a vast amount to learn, and, as a doctor, you have to work some pretty difficult hours, balancing clinical work against*

administrative, management and regulatory burdens, while still finding time to teach and to keep your own skills up to date. And it can be emotionally draining.

It's a hectic and challenging life, but the more I learn about it, the more I'd love to do it. I think I have both the academic aptitude and social skills to learn and thrive in that kind of environment. Being a doctor is definitely what I want to do.

Potential pitfalls lie in wait for the unwary candidate. Here are some answer no-nos:

- ✔ Avoid answers that imply a purely academic perspective. For instance, getting straight As or A*s isn't a reason to apply to medical school. It may be a reason to include medicine as one of several different options when narrowing the field of degrees down, but that's not the same thing as being a reason for actually choosing it.

- ✔ Don't focus on the financial or social rewards of medicine. Applying to study medicine because it offers a job with moderately high social status and a comfortable income stream is unlikely to score well with interviewers, even though such considerations inevitably form some part of everyone's practical decision-making.

- ✔ Refrain from saying that you're choosing medicine because you don't like the idea of going into politics or becoming a barrister, or that you want to be a doctor because other family members already are.

Very few candidates explicitly make these mistakes, but many inadvertently imply these things. For instance, saying 'my father is a doctor, so I've grown up seeing what being a doctor requires' may not directly suggest that you want to be a doctor because of your father, but it seeds that thought in an interviewer's mind. If you want to demonstrate that you have a good understanding of the duties and demands of the profession, do so by giving examples from your work experience, not through citing family members.

Detailing your work experience: 'How have you tested your commitment to medicine?'

You may be asked this question if you haven't already covered your work experience through a previous question. Interviewers can also ask it explicitly: 'Tell me about your work experience' or 'What steps have you taken to prove that medicine is right for you?'. All these variants check for enthusiasm, drive and a realistic understanding of a career in medicine.

Use this question as an opportunity to showcase a few highlights of your work experience and what you learned from them.

 For this question, quality matters far more than quantity. Ten items of work experience where you sat idly in a clinic learning little counts for far less than two items of work experience that you can discuss practically and weigh up with the interviewers.

If interviewers phrase the question sufficiently broadly, also include other essential elements of the pre-application process, such as talking to medical students and practising doctors, going to university open days, and perhaps attending courses or seminars and reading up about medical issues.

 Show balance in your discussion of your work experience: like any job, medicine isn't relentlessly blissful. Discussing the practical strains of the job while still showing optimism and enthusiasm very much counts in your favour.

 Take a look at the following sample answer and identify why it works.

I thought carefully before applying to medical school. I asked several doctors what they thought about the job. The consensus was that it's a profession in flux and under a lot of pressure, but that medicine is still a uniquely enjoyable career. They thought I'd do well as a doctor.

I went to several open days, including one at this university, and was impressed by the course structure. I like the idea of a strongly demarcated pre-clinical course before moving on to clinical work later; it appeals to how I like to think about life. Get the right foundations first, and then build on that.

I've had work experience in different settings, from a tertiary referral centre to my local GP surgery. They're all very different and I learned a lot, especially about how to balance clinical work against the other aspects of being a doctor, like teaching, research and management.

The experience that really sticks in my mind is a more personal one, though. I was shadowing a physician who had to tell a patient that she had cancer. She was such a bright and vivacious lady, and you could see in her eyes that her world was collapsing around her as the doctor broke the bad news.

He was very sympathetic in his approach and managed to steer the consultation on to what could be done next in a sensitive but still efficient manner. I was very impressed at his ability to think strategically at the same time as being emotionally present in order to help her feel supported. Getting that balance right is a really high-level skill, and I want to help people in a similar way.

Many interviewees realise this question is largely about work experience, but they begin reeling off a long list of what they did. Interviewers are interested in why that work experience convinced you that medicine was the right career for you and that you would make a good doctor. A long list doesn't convince them of that; discuss and explain your work experience instead.

Understanding your role as a doctor: 'Why didn't you choose nursing?'

Candidates often panic and answer this question badly, but the interviewers aren't trying to tell you to apply for a nursing degree. They just want to see that you understand what separates medicine from nursing, and that you can work effectively in a team with other health professionals.

Good answers focus first on the positive work nurses do: they're highly trained professionals in their own regard, and work alongside doctors and other health professionals to deliver high-quality care for patients. Recognise that their role is changing and expanding. For instance, nurses are found in ward, team and trust management roles and can possess (somewhat limited) prescribing powers.

Go on, however, to say that you know that differences exist between nurses and doctors. Doctors still have longer and more academic training than nurses, despite some narrowing of the gap. Doctors have the final responsibility for patient care and that often means they help drive the decision-making process forward.

Medicine therefore appeals to those who want to take on the pressure of this responsibility and work with a team of professionals to implement good patient care.

The priority is to avoid accidentally disrespecting nurses with your answer, thereby indicating that you'd struggle to work with them.

Explaining your choice of school: 'Why have you applied here?'

Universities are eager to know that you want to study at their institution. Every medical school is different and they tend to choose students who fit their way of teaching and overall ethos. As a result, you need to research your choices carefully and, if asked about it at interview, be able to explain your research process.

A logical starting point is to talk about the institution's website/prospectus and your open-day visits, discussing the course structure and the school's academic reputation. Explain how and why it suits your learning style, going on to mention the atmosphere and general setting.

Avoid glib answers involving elements such as pretty buildings, low rents or proximity to your home.

Knowing yourself: 'What's your main weakness?'

This question is a tired cliché. Unfortunately it still appears in interviews, and even more unfortunately, most candidates' answers are equally clichéd. Its purpose is to test your self-knowledge; to check that you recognise your limitations and how to progress beyond them.

The best answers discuss a genuine area of weakness, and then explain how you're addressing it:

> I enjoy talking to people and have found that I'm very good at negotiating with them and convincing them that my plans are for the best. The flipside of that is that I can sometimes inadvertently browbeat people through force of argument.

> To compensate for that, I've learned that it's sometimes important to take a step back and let people make their own informed decisions, even if I think they're wrong, and try to ensure that no harm results if their decision proves incorrect.

> It's not always easy to do this, but I've found it can result in better long-term outcomes and better communication.

Avoid the trap of trotting out predictable answers such as 'I'm a perfectionist' or superficial statements like 'I eat too much junk food'. And definitely don't say things that raise serious questions about your suitability for a career in medicine, such as 'I'm too careless' or 'I don't like talking to people'.

Understanding a Medical Career

As well as getting a read on your personality and skills, interviewers frequently check that you understand what a career in medicine involves. Some of that is covered by the questions we discuss in the earlier section 'Talking About Yourself', but interviewers can also ask you about it more directly.

Researching doctors' tasks: 'What does a doctor do in an average week?'

Some prospective medical students think that all a doctor does is treat patients. That's obviously an important part of the job, but doctors are also involved in other activities that enable them to do their clinical work better and deliver care more efficiently. As well as treating patients with medication or surgery, doctors:

- **Promote health:** This advice on healthy living reduces the chances of patients getting ill in the first place.

- **Counsel:** This helps patients cope with the impact of illness. Doctors need good communication skills to counsel patients in the immediate aftermath of diagnosis and may refer them to dedicated counselling services.

- **Continue their professional development:** By attending lectures, conferences and other activities, doctors keep their skills up to date.

- **Teach others:** For example, medical students or junior doctors.

- **Manage:** Taking part in management and clinical governance activities ensures that individual and trust practice meet the accepted best standards of care.

And, of course, doctors also maintain a life outside of medicine!

Don't just focus on clinical work. This can make you look naive as doctors have to do much more than just that. Balance the vital importance of clinical care against the many other demands on a doctor's time.

Thinking about your chosen career: 'What makes a good doctor?'

The General Medical Council (GMC) produces a useful document called *Good Medical Practice*, which covers the duties of a doctor and what makes for a good one.

Although the current version dates from 2006, and is currently being revised with a view to publication by early 2013, we doubt that the revised version will massively deviate from the current content. Therefore, you can use it as a spine around which to build your answer to this interview question. Such an approach shows a high level of familiarity with the topic and usually scores well with interviewers.

Good Medical Practice currently states that as a doctor you need to:

✔ Make the care of your patient your first concern.

✔ Provide a good standard of practice and care, which involves:

- Keeping your professional knowledge/skills up to date.

- Working within the limits of your competence.

- Working with colleagues to best serve patients' interests.

✔ Work in partnership with patients, including:

- Listening to patients and responding to their concerns and preferences.

- Giving patients the information they want or need in a way they can understand.

- Respecting patients' right to reach decisions with you about their treatment and care.

- Supporting patients in caring for themselves to improve and maintain their health.

✔ Be honest and open and act with integrity.

Don't rush into giving a glib, one-sentence answer. This question is about having a strong sense of ethics and an ability to reflect on life. It raises important issues and these should be given due weight in your answer.

Demonstrating that you're well informed: 'What are the good and bad points of being a doctor?'

We cover some of the pros and cons of a career in medicine in Chapter 1. But if you're asked this question in an interview, focus on positives such as the variety, challenge and satisfaction of the job, and the negatives of stress and systemic problems of working in medicine. Then go on to say how you'd cope with those challenges.

A sample answer may be:

One of the best things about being a doctor is the sheer variety involved. While you may have a typical weekly schedule, it's common not to know exactly what you'll have to manage on any given day and you meet a real cross-section of the public. When you combine that unpredictability with the opportunity to make a real difference to people in distress, you have a genuinely exciting and interesting career.

Of course, you have to work very hard both to qualify as a doctor and then when you're actually doing the job. The hours are less long than they used to be, but they're just as antisocial, if not more so, with lots of nights and weekend shifts. But I think keeping your overall reasons for being a doctor in mind should go a long way to keeping motivation high.

I know that doctors often struggle with the quantity of paperwork and bureaucracy involved in modern healthcare. It's meant to ensure efficient and high quality practice, but many health professionals feel that a lot of it misses the point. I hope at some stage to be involved in working with others to help refine and improve the system.

Medicine can be emotionally draining at times, too. Good supervision and maintaining a good work-life balance should help reduce the stress.

Avoid answers that include the financial rewards or which hint at laziness regarding the work involved.

Thinking around Scenarios

As part of their work doctors encounter some pretty unusual situations, and interviewers want to check whether you have the right skills to cope with them. They may question you about situations you've handled in the past, or ask you how you'd behave in hypothetical future scenarios. This approach is sometimes called *behavioural interviewing*.

You have to answer these questions crisply and concisely, with a minimum of waffle. Ensure that each answer takes you 2–3 minutes to relate at most.

Displaying the right stuff: 'Give an example of a time when you demonstrated. . .'

The questioner finishes this question by asking about a specific skill. Although this behaviour can be anything, common areas include:

- ✔ Communication skills
- ✔ Initiative and creativity
- ✔ Organisational skills
- ✔ Rational thinking
- ✔ Team work and leadership

This type of question often puts students off. It requires a combination of lateral and logical thinking that's quite difficult to pull off in an interview setting. Fortunately, you can prepare well for this question by doing the heavy lifting in advance.

Think of a small handful of situations that you've been in where you had to use these kinds of skills. Try to come up with three or four scenarios where more than one skill was used, so that you can spin them easily in whatever direction the questioner wants.

If you can't think of any pertinent scenarios, try breaking your experiences down into different domains. Think about your school life, extracurricular activities, family life and your friends. You're bound to come up with some situations that required non-academic skills. Look at the brainstorming ideas we ask you to draw up in Chapter 4, or at your personal statement (see Chapter 5), for some ideas.

When you've identified the scenario, you need to explain how you used the skill. Instead of improvising a structure on the day, take advantage of a well-known system called the *STAR technique*. STAR stands for Situation, Task, Action, Result and is an excellent way to describe your actions when tackling any problem:

- ✔ **Situation:** Describe the situation and its context. Who was involved, where was this and when did it happen?

- ✔ **Task:** What was your objective? Don't waffle around this; be definitive.

- ✔ **Action:** What did you do? Be specific. Describe what you did and why you did it.

- ✔ **Result:** What happened? What did you learn? If the outcome was negative, explain what you'd do in a similar situation next time.

Here's a sample answer using the STAR technique for an interview question asking you to describe a situation where you had to demonstrate good organisational skills:

Last year, I was asked to arrange a charity auction for our local hospice. I was given a date when it would be held, and a venue, but I needed to obtain the lots, find an auctioneer and arrange publicity.

I therefore rang around and visited a range of local businesses to ask them to donate items to be auctioned. Fortunately, they were all quite generous. A local cafe agreed to provide some free catering in lieu of offering a prize, provided we acknowledged their help, which was great.

A friend of a friend knew a local TV presenter and she was happy to come along and be the auctioneer. Once that was arranged, the charity agreed to fund the printing of leaflets and posters to advertise the auction, and I spoke to a journalist at the local newspaper who published a piece. Our local radio station also agreed to mention it in passing, which was really useful in drumming up awareness.

On the day, despite a few nerves, everything went pretty well. We raised over £5,500 for the charity, which they said was more than they expected. If I had to do it again, I'd probably be a little more ambitious in terms of venue and lots as there seemed to be a great deal of goodwill towards the event.

This type of question is frequently answered very badly. Candidates either panic and say nothing, or start a very rambling and confusing story. Stick to a clear and consistent structure like the STAR technique to avoid falling into these traps.

Coping with tricky events: 'How would you deal with. . . ?'

This question is similar to the one in the preceding section except that, instead of asking you to describe a historical situation, it involves considering a hypothetical scenario. For example, interviewers may ask you how you'd cope with an angry patient, a colleague who turns up to work intoxicated, explaining to a patient that he has a terminal illness, discussing how to administer healthcare budget cuts fairly or more abstract topics that touch on similar ethical issues, such as choosing who to save in the event of a nuclear apocalypse.

You can use the STAR technique from the preceding section to answer this question well, but be sure to flag up and address any specific risks to yourself or others right at the start. Here's a sample answer for dealing with an angry patient:

> *If I were dealing with an angry patient, my first priority would be to ensure the situation was safe. If he was physically aggressive, or I feared he would become so, I'd ensure that hospital security was called and that no vulnerable people were nearby. I wouldn't approach him if the situation was unsafe, or at risk of becoming so.*

> *If he were simply angry but not aggressive, I'd want to calmly listen to him and try to find out the underlying problem. Initially I'd like to let him vent his anger, in the hope this would take some of the immediate heat out of the situation. I'd avoid raising my own voice and acknowledge any mistakes that may have been made, as well as empathise – as far as is reasonable – with his feelings.*

> *If possible, I'd try to come up with a mutually agreeable plan for resolving the underlying reasons for his anger and ensure that someone keeps in touch with him to check that the problem is being resolved.*

Beware of giving a vague and rambling answer. Use a structure like the STAR technique to give your answer a clear narrative progression.

Tackling controversies: 'What do you think about. . .?'

This question asks your opinion about a controversial ethical issue or newsworthy healthcare topic.

Interviewers don't really care what your opinion is; they want to see you demonstrate a rational, sensible approach to thinking around contentious topics.

In Chapter 13 we discuss some topics that candidates are frequently asked about, but you can't prepare for every issue under the sun. Instead you have to think logically. Here's a good approach to take:

1. **Acknowledge the difficult, controversial and emotive nature of the topic.** If easy answers were available, the issue wouldn't be worth talking about.

2. **Summarise the arguments on one side of the debate, before doing the same for the other side.** If the question has a legal dimension and you know the current legislation, be sure to explain it.

3. **Venture a tentative personal opinion.** We suggest that you don't say anything too controversial or that raises questions about your ethical perspective.

Candidates frequently rush to judgement and begin their answer with an absolute statement that is often unsupported by evidence or rational argument. This comes across badly because controversial issues are controversial precisely because there's no right answer. Demonstrate thoughtfulness and an ability to see both sides of the argument before offering a balanced conclusion.

Revealing your determination: 'What will you do if you don't get in?'

Being asked what you'll do if you don't get into medical school can be frightening, but just remember that it doesn't imply that the interviewers have decided to reject you! They simply want to test your commitment to a career in medicine.

A good response is to accept that you'd be disappointed because you worked hard at your application, but that you'd then try to get feedback from medical schools and remedy whatever deficits they brought up.

Preparing a contingency plan for reapplying the following year that you can describe to interviewers is also worthwhile. Ideally, detail how you'd make the most of the resulting gap year to improve your skills and strengthen your application.

Don't fall into the trap of being too self-effacing. Saying something like, 'it was always a long shot so I wouldn't be too disappointed' makes you sound weak and uncommitted.

Speaking and listening well: 'What are good communication skills?'

Good communication is very simple: it involves talking and listening! Both are important, of course, but in practice most people forget about the listening part. Good listeners:

- ✔ Display warmth and empathy.
- ✔ Listen quietly, checking they've understood what the other person is saying.
- ✔ Ask gently probing questions to get further information.
- ✔ Reflect on what's been said to try to get to deeper truths.

When they talk, good communicators speak clearly and unambiguously in order to get their message across concisely. They check the other person has understood, avoid jargon and may use non-verbal communication methods such as diagrams or models to explain difficult concepts.

No doubt you realise that as well as providing a structure for explaining good communication skills, the above paragraphs also detail the very skills you need to deploy to perform well in an interview.

Expecting the unexpected: The uncommon question

Some questions, especially in Oxbridge interviews, are on such obscure topics that preparing for them is quite impossible. These questions are deliberately designed to be unexpected, because the interviewers are testing your intellectual alacrity and adaptability as well as your ability to cope with pressure. Examples include questions as diverse as 'What is truth?' or 'What's the length of the coastline of Great Britain?' (see the nearby sidebar 'How long is Britain's coastline?').

How long is Britain's coastline?

The coastline problem has many potential solutions, from going out and practically measuring it with a rolling wheel or laser, to using ordnance survey maps to calculate it.

Another way is to simplify the geometry of Britain into polygons (such as rectangles and triangles) and then measure the sides of that simplified diagram. This approach generates only an approximate result but so do the other methods just mentioned. The more complex the polygons, the closer the diagram approximates reality and the more accurate the measurement.

This method of measurement is conceptually equivalent to using rulers of different lengths: a yardstick naturally yields a more approximate result when measuring a complex shape than a small ruler does. This principle has an interesting consequence: the smaller the measuring device, the longer the coastline of Britain seems to be. In fact, if you had an infinitely small ruler, you'd have an infinitely long coastline, which would seem like a ridiculous proposition to a practical-minded surveyor. But not so to the mathematician Bertram Mandelbrot, the father of Fractal Theory.

Essentially, as with many natural phenomena, the coastline of Britain is a giant fractal problem: the closer you zoom into any portion of coast, the more detail emerges. Measuring its length accurately is impossible unless you first agree on a certain fixed degree of precision.

Of course, universities don't expect you to know all of this background detail. They want to see that you can think on your feet. Faced with this coastline problem, a good candidate would point out the difficulty of the task and highlight a few different methods of measurement. An outstanding candidate would note that each method would have a different level of precision, and that the level of precision required therefore needs to be predetermined.

This type of question is very good at discriminating between good and exceptional candidates by allowing them to explore the problem right up to the limit of their problem-solving abilities.

Here are some tips:

- ✔ Take an initial moment to check the question with the interviewer and think about how you're going to approach it.

- ✔ Be relentlessly logical, breaking the problem down into more manageable component parts.

- ✔ If in doubt, approach the problem conceptually, exploring it from different philosophical angles: for example, legal, ethical, practical, financial, political, scientific and so on.

✔ Be circumspect, reserving and qualifying judgement where needed. However, be clear that these reservations aren't down to indecision but to the fundamental uncertainty surrounding the problem.

✔ Above all, don't flap! Many candidates do; if you simply keep cool, you're already miles ahead of the competition.

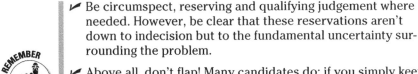

Questioning the Questioners: 'Do You Have Any Questions for Us?'

Almost every interview ends with this question. You don't need to ask anything; simply stating, 'No, thank you,' smiling and saying goodbye when they subsequently wave you away is perfectly acceptable.

If you have a genuine area of interest, however, this is an opportunity to ask about it, as well as a chance to follow-up on an earlier question, especially if you feel you didn't answer it well. You can ask what the answer was, or how you could best have approached it.

Don't ask something trivial for the sake of it or something you should already know from your research.

Chapter 13

Staying Current: Medical Topics You Need to Know About

. . . .

In This Chapter

▶ Looking at the NHS and medicine in the UK

▶ Familiarising yourself with ethical issues

. . . .

*I*n the UK, nearly all doctors start their careers in the National Health Service (NHS); indeed, many spend their entire working lives in it. Therefore, understanding life in the NHS is important because medical schools like to test that knowledge during interviews and also so you can decide whether it's a setting you're going to enjoy.

Medical school interviewers frequently ask your opinion on recent changes to the NHS and new advances in medicine. Partly, they're checking your enthusiasm and commitment to a career in medicine and partly they want to see that you can think intelligently around these issues. They may also give you a controversial ethical dilemma and ask your opinion. Remember that no easy answers exist to these dilemmas; interviewers are looking to hear a sensible and compassionate answer.

To help with your medical school interviews, we provide information about medicine in the UK and a few medical ethical issues. Exhaustive detail on all these topics is beyond the scope of this book, but we give you a great jumping off point for further independent research. By discussing these issues, you can begin to see how doctors approach decision-making. Developing that mindset helps you do well in interviews and throughout medical school.

Keeping up to date is possible by reading the health sections of broadsheet newspapers and their online equivalents like the NHS Behind the Headlines: www.nhs.uk/news/Pages/NewsIndex. aspx. But to make life easier for you, we maintain a news-aggregating at http://GetIntoMedicineUK.com, which highlights interesting healthcare-related stories and suggests areas to think about in order to understand their implications more fully.

Understanding How the NHS Works

The history, nature and workings of the NHS – which currently provides the vast majority of its treatments free at the point of use – may crop up in medical school interviews. The NHS provides a broad range of healthcare services to everyone in the UK. To help your interview preparation, we split the information we provide into factual details about its formation and organisation and more practical aspects of life as an NHS doctor.

Getting to grips with NHS facts

The NHS is a vast, hugely complex organisation. Virtually every doctor in the UK works in the NHS at some point, and even those that subsequently work in the private sector will still interact with NHS hospitals and staff. It arouses strong passions among professionals and the general public. The more you know about its history, development and management, the better prepared you are for any questions about it during your medical school interview.

Knowing its history

The NHS was founded in 1948 by the post-war government but its origin lies in the Second World War. Before that, some healthcare was provided free of charge to the poor by a mix of charitable institutions and teaching hospitals but necessarily on a haphazard basis. The middle classes had access to health insurance and the wealthy paid for medical care.

During the war, a centralised state-run medical service directly employed medical staff to treat the injured. The general strain of the war effort on national resources led to a broad feeling that an effort should be made to distribute this service evenly to all people. The Liberal politician Lord Beveridge published a famous report in 1942 suggesting the creation of a national health service funded from general taxation and run by central government.

After the war, this proposal was taken up and in 1948 the NHS was founded, though not without considerable political difficulty and the need to pay substantial sums to hospitals and doctors to convince them to participate.

If asked about the role of NHS in the UK during an interview, a good starting point is to give a brief overview of its creation and the historical context surrounding it at that time. This section provides the bones around which you can flesh out a good answer.

Briefly recapping the history of the NHS also provides you with some precious thinking time if their question requires you to think about its current relevance to society.

Pondering spending pressures in the NHS

The initial NHS supporters accepted that it would be very expensive to set up, but they argued that over time costs would subside. This view was partly because the one-off capital expense of purchasing private hospitals would fade, but also due to the somewhat naive expectation that illness rates would fall. The belief was that if the general population had access to good quality healthcare, people across society would become healthier and fewer would need medical attention. In other words, the NHS would cost less because people wouldn't need it so much.

You can almost see the logic; at the time the NHS was founded, two major groups of patients were those suffering with war injuries and those with infectious diseases. With the war over, the idea was that the cohort of injured veterans would gradually fall away, and with the advent of seemingly magical industrially-produced antibiotics, infectious diseases could be eradicated.

Of course, these optimistic projections were short-lived. Although antibiotics certainly made a real difference to public health, unfortunately over time some pathogens began to develop resistance, necessitating more elaborate (and expensive) antimicrobial therapy.

More fundamentally, though infectious disease rates fell, people still have to die of something. If they don't die of infection or trauma, they suffer from longer-term, chronic illnesses instead. Britain's biggest killers today are cancer, and cardiovascular, neurological, endocrine or degenerative conditions. These conditions can often be partly contained for many years but, unfortunately, outright cure is rare. So they're much more expensive to treat than acute illnesses that result in rapid cure or kill. The country's ageing population means more chronic illness and therefore more expense.

Shifting cultural expectations

In 1948, people were so grateful to have freely available healthcare that they accepted any quality. Today, people are accustomed to the NHS and expect world-class healthcare, which for the reasons we describe in this section is very expensive to provide.

Indeed, many experts argue that healthcare demand grows over time, requiring an ever-increasing proportion of national wealth. The economies of almost all countries bear witness to this ratcheting effect.

In addition, medicine is far more sophisticated than in 1948. For example, devices – such as magnetic resonance imaging (MRI) scanners – and medicines – such as antiretroviral combination therapy for HIV – are wonderful innovations that improve lives. But they're phenomenally expensive compared to the diagnostic and therapeutic interventions available at the time of the founding of the NHS. The nearby sidebar 'Shifting cultural expectations' describes how these expenses are complicated by the nation's expectations.

In an effort to contain rising costs, successive governments of all political stripes have reorganised the NHS in an attempt to increase efficiency and deliver more healthcare per pound spent.

 The NHS is responsible for about one pound out of every five spent by the British government. Despite that, it has experienced spending pressures almost from its creation. You may be asked to discuss that level of spending in an interview. A good answer may start with a discussion of why healthcare generally is so expensive, using some of the points raised in this section, and then reviewing whether the NHS represents good value for money compared to other healthcare systems.

Rationing in the NHS

The NHS has always supplied rationed care, for the simple reason that the demand for healthcare exceeds supply. The NHS doesn't select by the ability to pay, and so it has to ration care in other ways. Sometimes this is done openly, though all politicians shy away from using the word 'rationing'. Frequently, it happens surreptitiously. For example, waiting lists for appointments or operations are subtle forms of rationing. They match the delivery of healthcare to the resources available.

To make rationing more transparent, in 2005 the National Institute for Health and Clinical Excellence (NICE) was founded to review new treatments and decide which should be provided on the NHS. Crucially, one criterion is cost-effectiveness. Even if a treatment works, if it's too expensive, NICE rejects its use.

Comparing different treatments is difficult and controversial. Some techniques try to measure how many potential healthy years of life a treatment offers a patient, valuing treatments that bestow more good years over treatments that offer only a few. This is the basis of the Quality Adjusted Life Year (QALY) approach. As you may well have spotted, used in isolation QALY systematically biases care away from the elderly and towards children because they always gain more years from successful treatment.

Of course, NICE uses a range of different methods to reach recommendations, but controversy is inevitable and several NICE decisions have been reversed by sustained public campaigns, for example in the case of some Alzheimer disease and breast cancer drugs. This raises the possibility that groups capable of organising themselves politically can pressurise NICE, so biasing healthcare towards the vocal and self-assertive middle classes instead of the most vulnerable.

NHS rationing will always need to exist in one form or another because tax revenue is ultimately finite. Another way of balancing supply and demand is to reorganise healthcare to create more supply. This latter argument underpins the ideology behind the most recent reorganisation of the NHS, which we describe in the following section.

Think about these issues of financing and rationing. Should future governments increase general taxation to relieve the NHS's pressures or is this a futile endeavour? How do other healthcare systems around the world balance these demands? Answering these questions in a politically-balanced way shows maturity and perspective. When faced with such complex questions, start by acknowledging the difficulty and sensitivity of the topic. Then explore the issue from as many different angles as you can think of: economic, sentimental, political, legal, philosophical. For example, what is the fairest way of dividing up resources? What does 'fair' really mean?

Explaining the Health and Social Care Act 2012

The Health and Social Care Act 2012 is now law. It has significant implications for the NHS and quite reasonably interviewers may ask your opinion of the changes. The Act is politically controversial and very broad in scope and no one expects you to have a comprehensive grasp of its detail. But if you can display knowledge of a basic outline of the changes, you're miles ahead of your competition trying to get into medical school.

Be cautious when developing and expressing your opinion; healthcare is a highly complex system and knowing how changes are going to pan out is extremely difficult.

The NHS is state-funded from the pool of money received by the Treasury in general taxation. Before the 2012 Act, management was organised into 10 regional Strategic Health Authorities (SHAs), with about 150 Primary Care Trusts (PCTs) underneath, covering smaller regional subdivisions. PCT executive boards generally had some elected representation from local primary care providers, such as GPs. PCTs *commissioned* (that is, bought) the services they needed for their patients from other branches of the NHS such as hospital trusts, GPs, mental health trusts and ambulance trusts. PCTs also commissioned services from the private, non-profit and voluntary sectors, but technical aspects of the commissioning process made it very difficult for a non-NHS body to win a contract if an existing NHS service already provided that care.

Based on the money they received from their contracts with PCTs, all the above groups provided care for the patient groups they were contracted to serve.

The 2012 Act contains a number of important changes to this system. Here are several of the main points:

- ✔ The SHA and PCT layers of management are removed and in their place is a slimmed-down layer of regional strategic representation, which no longer has commissioning powers.

- ✔ Over 200 Clinical Commissioning Groups (CCGs), comprising primarily GPs but also including some other local healthcare practitioners (such as hospital doctors, nurses and so on), now commission services. The inclusion of these latter groups into CCGs was a compromise by the government.

- ✔ As with the old PCTs, CCGs can commission services from the private, non-profit and voluntary sectors. However, technical changes (the 'any qualified provider' clause) in the commissioning process substantially increase the likelihood that these sectors will demonstrate that they can provide the needed care. They're likely to win contracts away from NHS organisations if they can meet the need at a lower cost.

- ✔ GPs (and some specialist services) aren't funded by CCGs, but directly from government.

✔ Based on the money they receive centrally (in the case of GPs) or from CCGs (in the case of other organisations), these groups now provide care to the patient groups they're contracted to serve.

With the 2012 Act, the government's stated aims are as follows:

✔ NHS spending continues to be funded from general taxation.

✔ The percentage of its expenditure on non-NHS (private, non-profit, voluntary) sectors is likely to increase, although this isn't certain. This change should increase efficiency through more competition between qualified providers for contracts. The NHS will be able to provide more healthcare per pound spent.

✔ The Act will fuel the development of a more diverse healthcare ecosystem that can better meet the needs of individual patients, compared to a monolithic NHS service defined centrally.

✔ Healthcare practitioners representing smaller, more local, groups of patients will commission NHS services. This may make commissioning more responsive to local care needs.

The counter-arguments include:

✔ On an ideological level, some people oppose any expansion of the involvement of non-NHS organisations in the delivery of NHS care, because they feel that the NHS should be a public organisation where healthcare is provided by public servants (not employees of private, non-profit or voluntary organisations). Reasons for this position vary from the political to the ethical, depending on the individual.

✔ Some object to the changes on practical grounds, saying that large-scale changes add a disruptive burden to the delivery of care during a financially difficult time. They suggest that the changes are a distraction, paradoxically increasing short-term costs and inefficiency resulting from the need to manage the reorganisation.

✔ Other people fear that a more diverse healthcare ecosystem will eventually lead to an expansion of the private sector, attracting healthcare practitioners into it rather than the NHS.

If asked about the Act in an interview, a wise course of action is to acknowledge the controversial nature of the changes, and use the STAR approach that we outline in Chapter 12 to explain the problem, the nature of the Act and the potential results, arguing first from one side of the debate and then the other. Finally, wrap up by acknowledging that the outcome is uncertain.

If you want to, you can also offer a tentative opinion about which outcomes are more likely. But avoid being overly political in your answer; you don't know the interviewers' opinion, and they're more interested in your understanding than your political allegiance.

Computing in healthcare

In the earlier section 'Pondering spending pressures in the NHS', we mention the cost of general technological innovation in healthcare. Well, another area that's similarly challenged is computing. The infrastructure of the NHS is increasingly computerised, from appointment systems to record-keeping, billing and accountancy.

The NHS adopted information technology (IT) piecemeal in the 1980s and 1990s. Different GP surgeries and hospitals had their own bespoke systems and none of them talked to each other. Eventually, government decided that a good idea would be to develop a single, unified IT framework for the NHS in order to benefit from improved communication and other efficiencies. This was the aim of the National Programme for IT (NPfIT), but unfortunately the task was larger and more complicated than anyone expected. By the time the project was terminated, costs spiralled from £1 billion to over £12 billion, with no completion date in sight.

A single IT framework is a good idea, but the costs became so high that the project was undeliverable.

The hope now is that enough of the hard groundwork has been done to allow a final merging of systems over time in a slower, more organic way. One crucial completed element was the Choose & Book system necessary to allow different providers to compete for patients, and to account for the money that accompanies them from their CCG (which we define in the preceding section).

Interviewers may question you on the use of technology in the NHS. One line of questioning would be to check your familiarity with projects like the NPfIT (National Project for Information Technology) and then go on to ask you whether the NHS should invest in information technology. A sensible approach would be to discuss the advantages, both in terms of patient care and freeing up time and money to devote to that care. Then balance that with a review of the cost and complexity of implementing large-scale technology projects. You may want to conclude by offering your thoughts as to how approach judging the relative strength of the two sides of the argument.

Working in the NHS

Medical schools like to know that prospective students have a rough idea of what life is like in the NHS. The information in this section reviews some practical aspects such as the hours you're going to be expected to work and the NHS career structure. Incorporating this practical knowledge into answers to questions about whether you understand the reality of life as a doctor, demonstrates to interviewers that you have a good insight into your application decision.

Putting in the hours

In the past, doctors worked gruelling hours. In our first jobs, we worked 80+ hour weeks and the cohort before us worked 100+ hours! Today, the European Working Time Directive (EWTD) limits doctors' hours to 48 per week. The system needed to change; it wasn't reasonable for doctors to work such long hours. Dangerous mistakes happened.

Medicine, however, is always going to be a 24-hour service. The result of doctors working fewer hours is that fewer are available at any given time, and doctors need to work more antisocial patterns such as weeks of night shifts.

Junior doctors also need to learn their trade. With the reduction in hours comes a reduction in informal learning experiences through the traditional apprenticeship model of working alongside senior colleagues and picking up techniques and information. Therefore, more formalised teaching sessions now take place, with varying degrees of success in engaging junior doctors and delivering high-quality educational experiences. Young surgeons in particular have struggled to replace the operating theatre time lost by the introduction of the EWTD.

The reduction in the number of doctors available in hospital at any given time places strains on both day and night shifts. During the day, consultants increasingly lead teams with juniors that are absent for weeks at a time on nights, which can cause a fragmented and unhappy team. At nights, a skeleton team of doctors has to work across disciplinary boundaries because not every speciality always has a senior member at work. The system can even lead to the odd situation of a junior doctor on shift being more familiar with a particular procedure than the senior meant to be supervising her.

The potential problems associated with staffing a hospital at night haven't yet been solved. Any long-term solution is likely to include consultants working the same antisocial working patterns as their juniors, something unlikely to please those who thought they'd already paid their dues of long hours! Whether such a move results in senior doctors choosing to retire early, or going to work in the private sector where less such pressures exist, is yet to be seen.

The issue of doctors' working hours is complex and contentious. If interviewers raise the subject, use the information in this section to frame the current challenges to demonstrate awareness of the nuances of the argument.

Training after you're a doctor

All new doctors are provisionally registered with the General Medical Council (GMC). GMC provisional registration allows you to apply for Foundation Year 1 (FY1) posts. After FY1 is a second Foundation Year (FY2). Both FY1 and FY2 are rotations across a number of different specialities. You then apply to train in the speciality of your choice, the field of medicine that you'll practise after completing speciality training.

Doctors in training are Specialty Registrars (StRs), with the individual years of training numbered, for example, ST1, ST2 and so on. Training is often split between Core and Higher years, and in some specialities Core Trainees are given their own alphanumeric title, such as CT1, CT2 and CT3. In these specialities, Higher Trainees begin at the ST4 grade. In Core training you work towards passing your Royal College membership exams and in your Higher years you gain the experience to practise as a consultant.

GP trainees work within an analogous General Practice Vocational Training Scheme (GPVTS) while learning to become fully-fledged GPs.

In total, a typical doctor spends two years in Foundation grades and about six as an StR, for a total postgraduate training of eight years as a minimum before becoming a consultant. GP training is slightly shorter at a minimum of five years.

You'll still hear doctors, patients and other healthcare staff use terms such as Pre-Registration House Officer (PRHO), Senior House Officer (SHO) and Specialist Registrar (SpR). In fact, these titles are outdated terms for junior doctor posts that were phased out in 2007, when medical training went through a traumatic upheaval. PRHO corresponds roughly to Foundation, SHO to Core and SpR to Higher training.

The 2007 upheaval resulted in a lot of resentment by large swathes of the profession, especially juniors, who had to reapply for their own jobs. It embodied a longer-term fear that the profession is losing its autonomy and vocational nature and becoming more routine and managed.

Although probably true, scope still exists for finding a niche that suits your personality if you look hard enough and have the necessary talent. In addition, more recent changes to the healthcare system may make this easier through the development of a broader range of healthcare providers to work for.

If asked about your future career plans, it's fine to make a general statement about whether a hospital or GP setting appeals to you more. Make it clear that, at your stage, you're looking forward to training in a range of settings in order to learn more about what they involve. Avoid being too definite about which subspeciality you want to work in, as it's common for medical students to change their mind during training and it can seem a little presumptive to be too specific at a very early stage.

Certainly, avoid putting down any speciality in order to justify your choice of a different one.

Thinking about Ethical Problems

Interviewers love asking candidates about ethical dilemmas – and good candidates enjoy talking about them, because they offer the opportunity to demonstrate awareness of difficult issues and a rational approach to balancing conflicting demands. Each medical school applies its own policies around which topics are fair game for interviewers to raise, and which are too controversial to ask about. Although the range of potential topics is vast, certain subjects are perennial favourites and so we take a brief look at these areas.

Work on remembering some of the main arguments around each topic and practise discussing them. Also, think about how you'd balance the risks associated with making a decision in each case (for more on dealing with risk, check out the later section 'Accepting uncertainty').

Evaluating the arguments on abortion

Abortion – the deliberate termination of a pregnancy – is legal in mainland UK with minor differences in the rest of Great Britain, and a much more restrictive regime in Northern Ireland.

The Abortion Act 1967, as amended by the Human Fertilisation and Embryology Act 1990 (HFEA), governs abortion in mainland UK. It states that abortion can be carried out:

- ✔ At any time to save the woman's life or prevent grave permanent injury to her physical or mental health.

- ✔ Up to 24 weeks to avoid injury to physical or mental health to the mother.

- ✔ Up to 24 weeks to avoid injury to physical or mental health of existing children.

- ✔ If the child is likely to be severely physically or mentally handicapped.

The amendments of the HFEA reduced the term limit from an original 28 weeks to the current 24 weeks to reflect the advances of medical science in treating prematurely born infants.

Arguments in favour of legal abortion revolve around the following points:

- ✔ A woman should have autonomy: the right to decide what happens to her own body.

- ✔ Many women who want an abortion but can't access a legal one would instead find an illegal, riskier provider.

- ✔ A foetus isn't a fully-formed human being and therefore doesn't carry the same legal rights.

- ✔ Termination of a pregnancy is arguably preferable to bringing a child into a family that doesn't want it.

- ✔ Society shouldn't have to bear the burden of caring for an unwanted infant.

Arguments against legal abortion include:

- ✔ Even if the foetus isn't a fully-formed human being, it has the potential to become one, making abortion a form of murder.

- ✔ Abortion is psychologically painful for the mother and father.

✔ The practice may be open to abuse, for example serial abortions to achieve a desired genetic feature (so-called designer babies).

✔ Long adoption lists exist and preferably people should be given the opportunity to love an otherwise unwanted child instead of it being aborted.

✔ Other forms of birth control are available; the potential parents should have taken more responsibility for their actions.

Asking about the ethics of abortion isn't as common as it used to be, but it can still arise. Never give your personal opinion first; explain the ethical dilemma that surrounds it and outline the legal position. If you really want to give your own opinion, do so at the end, and give a reasoned argument to support it.

Examining euthanasia

Euthanasia (sometimes called 'mercy-killing') is taking action to deliberately terminate someone's life with the intent of ending their pain or suffering.

When discussing this issue, distinguish euthanasia from *assisted suicide,* which is enabling people to end their own life, for example by providing them with the tablets they need to overdose on.

Euthanasia and assisted suicide are currently illegal in the UK, although the legal waters are clouded by some high-profile cases in which the Crown Prosecution Service deemed that pursuing a prosecution wasn't in the public interest.

Arguments in favour of euthanasia and assisted suicide are that:

✔ People have the right to do what they want with their own bodies, including having their lives ended if they're suffering.

✔ It may prevent unnecessary suffering and preserves people's dignity.

✔ It frees up NHS resources.

✔ People can travel abroad to access legal assisted suicide clinics, for example in Switzerland. By not providing them in the UK, the system discriminates against those without the money to travel and pay.

Arguments against the practice include:

- ✔ Regulating it would be very difficult, making it potentially open to abuse by unethical doctors and selfish relatives.

- ✔ People may lack the legal capacity to make a valid decision or may have later changed their minds.

- ✔ People may feel pressured into it.

 High profile legal cases around assisted suicide and euthanasia have been in the news over recent years. Examples include those of Diane Pretty and Tony Nicklinson. Framing the legal and ethical argument around these cases shows that you take an active interest in medical ethics. You can read up on these cases from their newspaper and BBC online coverage.

Mulling over organ donation

The UK currently has an *opt-in system* for organ donors, which means that organ donation after death is voluntary and no consent is presumed. If you want to donate you use the Organ Donation Register, a national database, to indicate your consent. Nearly a third of the population carries a donor card confirming this fact. Still, the demand for organs is greater than the supply, and so the topic of an *opt-out* (presumed consent) system is regularly revisited. Under this system, unless you specifically indicate that you don't want your organs transplanted, consent would be presumed.

 It's most likely that under an opt-out system organ supply would increase, because opinion polling suggests that a larger percentage of the population is in favour of donating than carries a donor card. Against this argument, however, is the fact that many people are ill-informed and prone to inertia, especially about the topic of their own death. As a result, many people who wouldn't want to donate their organs may well fail to formally opt-out.

Another controversial topic related to organ donation is whether the donated organs should be offered to those whose lifestyles put their organs at risk. For example, how much responsibility do alcoholics have for damage to their livers?

The section on 'Considering changing lifestyles' later in this chapter revisits the complex interface between legislation, personal responsibility and available healthcare in more detail.

Interviewers don't expect candidates to be familiar with the details of organ transplantation surgery. Also, they won't ask you personal questions about your own organ donor status, so don't feel obliged to disclose that kind of private information.

Weighing up vivisection

Literally translated *vivisection* means 'cutting alive' and refers to the practice of carrying out experiments on animals. This action may be done to test the safety and tolerability of substances used in contact with the skin (for example, cosmetics), to test new medical treatments or to carry out research into how the body works.

Vivisection is legal but very highly regulated, with a number of safeguards to minimise the amount of experimentation and the level of suffering caused.

Arguments in favour of vivisection are:

- ✔ Animal testing can save human lives.
- ✔ Very tight regulations exist to reduce suffering; whatever remains is justified in the big picture of human progress.
- ✔ If these experiments aren't carried out in the UK, they would still occur, except in less well-regulated environments abroad. By doing this research within the UK, the overall amount of suffering to animals is therefore actually reduced.

Arguments against vivisection are:

- ✔ Subjecting animals to experimentation, regardless of the benefits to humans, is inherently cruel and unethical.
- ✔ Some people view an animal's life as being equal to a human's life.
- ✔ Animals can't give informed consent to the experiment.
- ✔ Many tests are unnecessary or repeated, especially as more suitable alternatives are now available, for example cell cultures and computer modelling.

Vivisection is a very emotive topic. Be careful of inadvertently offending an interviewer with a strong opinion either for or against it. Offer a balanced review of the facts around the topic instead.

Researching with stem cells

Humans have two main types of stem cell:

- ✔ **Adult stem cells** act as a repair system for the body.

- ✔ **Embryonic stem cells** are *pluripotent,* which means that they can differentiate into all the different specialised cell types.

Some medical researchers believe that treatments using stem cells can dramatically change medicine. A number of adult stem cell therapies already exist, for example bone marrow transplantation in leukaemia.

The hope is that the pluripotency of embryonic stem cells may help treat common conditions as varied as cancer, spinal cord injuries, multiple sclerosis, diabetes and more. For example, under careful control, they can potentially be used to regrow neural tissue or insulin-producing pancreatic cells. However, embryonic stem cell research remains very controversial to some people, especially when the cells are harvested from aborted foetuses or from excess in-vitro fertilisation embryos.

One possible alternative is the use of induced pluripotent stem cells (iPS cells), which are artificially derived from non-pluripotent cells by 'forcing' the expression of specific genes. They are similar to embryonic stem cells in many ways and may bypass the controversy around using those cells. However, at present whether they're completely equivalent to embryonic cells is unclear.

Stem cell research is complex and constantly changing. Don't be afraid to acknowledge that you have limited familiarity with its details. If interviewers ask you about it, they're going to be more interested in your understanding of its ethical implications.

Considering changing lifestyles

Not everyone lives a healthy lifestyle. Many people overeat, do too little exercise, smoke and drink too much alcohol. A controversial issue is how much the government should intervene in people's lifestyles to improve their health: after all, one person's 'nanny state' is another's compassionate or responsible society.

The issue is complicated by the fact that in the UK the NHS delivers most healthcare. Therefore, it costs the state (in other words, the country's taxpayers) to treat people who become ill because of their unhealthy lifestyle. As a result, some argue that the state has a right to limit healthcare to those who it feels aren't deliberately endangering their health. Using a similar argument, it would be fair to introduce legislation to prevent unhealthy behaviour.

The strongest argument against this approach is that people should fundamentally be free to decide how to live their lives; that is, they have a right to liberty and self-determination. Even on a purely financial level, one can argue that because everyone is potentially subject to taxation, everyone has a mutual obligation to fund the NHS and therefore a right to access its care.

In reality, the legislation is a complex muddle that tries to strike a balance between these extremes that reflects the wider view of society. For example, cigarettes are a legal product but subject to restrictions on use and hefty taxation; the money raised from tobacco taxes partly funds the NHS.

Thinking about these issues can help you decide for yourself what the balance between the individual and the state should be, which can help provide context to many of the ethical dilemmas in this section.

Accepting uncertainty

As well as the well-known controversial subjects that we cover in the preceding sections, we also want to talk about a more general issue that you'll face as a doctor: risk. Thinking about it now makes you a better candidate and, eventually, a better doctor.

Risk is part of the job. Doctors aren't omniscient and can't always predict the outcome of life and death situations. This reality makes life as a doctor stressful.

Most people are bad at analysing risk and become paralysed by uncertainty. Good doctors understand risk, assess it rapidly and competently, and communicate their understanding well to others. Finally, they take appropriate action.

At its most basic level, people's health is the sum total of all the different things going on in their body and mind. Change any variable and they feel better or worse. The intense complexity of the human body and the fact that medical science is imperfect, means that predicting the outcome of any given intervention (for example, drugs, surgery or simple conversation) with 100 per cent certainty is not possible. Instead, doctors assess a person carefully and then act in a way that minimises the harm while maximising benefit. The aphorism *primum non nocere* ('first do no harm'), sometimes attributed to the ancient Greek physician Hippocrates, underlines this duty.

As a doctor, your training gives you the confidence to act in the face of uncertainty even if that means taking the 'least-worst' option or sometimes choosing to do nothing. The problem is that patients and their families have much more difficulty accepting this logic. They're suffering and expect doctors always to make things better. Your job is to explain situations to them in a way they can understand.

You can, however, use various ways to contain risk. Perhaps the most important is to understand your own limitations and ask advice from more experienced people if you come up against those limits.

Knowledge is also important. Medical researchers have done a lot of work to figure out the best course of action in a tricky situation, but when no ideal course exists, good communication skills and excellent documentation of your reasoning can help explain the problem and protect you from litigation if a disappointing outcome results.

Over the past few decades, increasing rates of medical litigation have led to more defensive medical practice. *Defensive medicine* is where doctors order more investigations than strictly necessary, in order to be able to point to all those tests if something is missed. But every investigation carries risks, including the possibility of false negatives and false positives. By carrying out unnecessary tests, doctors risk creating more distress. Balancing the risk of a test against the risk of not requesting it can be an exceptionally fine decision. If a doctor is worried about litigation, that fear can tip her into favouring the test.

Thinking about medicine (and life) as a balancing of risks results in you developing robust decision-making, less second-guessing and better lateral thinking. Outcomes are improved and defensible.

When applying to medical school, such thinking helps you separate unimportant variables from important ones, for example in selecting a medical school or in deciding how to answer interview questions about complicated topics, such as the ones we cover in this chapter.

Chapter 14

Following the Interview

*A*fter your medical school interviews are over, the wait begins! Most schools take at least a couple of weeks to sift through their interview data and decide who gets an offer. UCAS contacts you when the university makes its decision. In this chapter you discover what happens during this tense period and how to plan your next steps – whatever the result. We provide advice if you receive offers and suggest options and guidance on coping if you miss out on a place.

Tracking Your Progress

UCAS allows you to track the progress of your application through your account with its website, via the appropriately named Track progress section. Staff members also contact you directly after universities have fully processed your application and made a decision about offering you a place.

Medical school decisions fall into one of three types:

✔ **Conditional offer:** This is by far the most common offer made by medical schools and means that even after accepting the place, you still have to reach the required standard in your exams in order to take up that place and start medical school. The standard varies among schools, but it's generally around three A grades at A-level, or equivalent.

✔ **Unconditional offer:** Much more rarely, universities make this type of offer, in which no specific grade requirements apply at A-level; the place is yours if you still want it. These offers were more common in the days when Oxford and Cambridge ran their own university-specific entrance exams.

✔ **Unsuccessful:** If a medical school decides that it's not the best fit for you, your application is marked in this way. All is not lost, though: flip to the later section 'Overcoming Obstacles' for your options.

Replying to Offers and Handling Acceptance

Medical schools process applications at different rates, which means that you get decisions from some universities before others. Although you can reply to offers straightaway, you don't need to make a decision on any offer until you know the outcome of all your applications.

Unless you absolutely have your heart set on a specific institution, wait until you know the decision of all the medical schools to which you applied before deciding which offer to accept.

After you accept an offer, the decision is irrevocable, so think carefully about all your offers before deciding.

When all your medical schools have made their decision, the clock starts ticking for you to make a final decision. The deadline date varies from year to year, and is also dependent on the date the final university makes its decision. As a guide, Table 14-1 shows the timeline for a sample year's application cycle.

Table 14-1	Decision Timeline for a Sample Year's Application Cycle
Last University Decision Date	*Reply Date Deadline*
31 March	8 May
9 May	6 June
7 June	27 June
18 July	25 July

Accepting offers

You have three potential reply options to each offer:

▮ ✔ **Decline:** You permanently turn down the offer of a place.

✔ **Firm acceptance:** You commit to taking up a place at that medical school. If the offer was conditional (see the earlier section 'Tracking Your Progress'), you still need to meet the required grades.

✔ **Insurance acceptance:** Your back-up choice. You commit to taking up the place at this institution if you meet its requirements, but don't meet the minimum grades for your firmly-accepted medical school.

You can have only one firm and one insurance acceptance.

You don't have to make an insurance acceptance at all, for example if you're absolutely certain that you're going to get the grades for your firm choice. Another reason not to have an insurance acceptance is if no difference exists in the grade requirement between your conditional offers, and you don't think that one institution offers some leeway if you only just miss out on the needed grades.

Nonetheless, you have nothing to lose by making an insurance acceptance alongside your firm one and we advise you to do so, just in case.

Going to medical school

If you receive an offer to study medicine and meet all your grade requirements . . . congratulations! Medical school is a hugely exciting time of life (both of us look back on it fondly). You're going to meet new people, form some enduring friendships, learn lots of interesting things, have fantastic experiences and generally embark on a new phase of life.

Attending medical school can also be a bit scary, especially at the start. At normal school, you're probably one of the best students in your class and used to getting top marks all the time. At medical school, however, you're studying alongside students of equal abilities and are never guaranteed pole position. That can be a bit of a shock to the system. Medical school exams can be tough and may represent the first time you've ever had to re-sit a test, which can also be a challenging experience. In addition, if you've never lived on your own, discovering how to manage your time by balancing fun activities with necessary study can be tricky.

Go into the experience with a positive and open outlook. Anticipate some tough times along with the good, and expect to have to work hard as well as enjoy yourself. Try not to take small setbacks to heart and keep focused on the big picture.

You're going to learn a lot about yourself and about what's really important in life. And at the end of the course, you're going to be a doctor and get to work in one of the most exciting, varied and privileged professions.

You're just starting out on a great adventure. Enjoy it!

Overcoming Obstacles

If you don't get any offers from medical schools after all the hard work you put into your application, you can feel like the world has ended. Everyone forgives you some gnashing of teeth and a few tears.

After the initial shock and disappointment, remind yourself that bad things can happen to good people through no fault of their own and that sometimes good candidates get no offers. Medical school applications are such a ridiculously competitive process that no guarantee of success ever exists.

Considering your next step

Your task in this unlucky situation is to plan what to do next.

The initial big decision is whether you really want to study medicine. Remember that (as we explain in Chapter 3) you used only four UCAS application slots for medical schools, and so a vacant fifth slot remains or (if you already applied for another course) you may still be waiting to hear back from one university. If you decide that medicine is absolutely the only option for you, this point is moot, but if you don't mind studying a different subject at undergraduate level, that fifth UCAS place becomes important.

The final UCAS application date is around the end of June, and so unsuccessful medical school applicants typically have a brief window of opportunity to add a fifth non-medical choice to their application. UCAS Extra (available through your existing application) offers a similar opportunity if you have no offers or acceptances after using all five slots. If you're eligible for UCAS Extra, a button appears on your Track screen when you log on to the website, allowing you to apply for another course.

If you pursue either of the above options and get an offer for another course, you still have a final chance to decide whether to accept it or not. If you do go on to study that course, towards the end of it you can think about whether to pursue the subject further or apply for graduate entry medicine (something we talk you through in Chapter 3).

If medicine feels like the only right choice for you, try to get feedback from the universities to which you applied. Frankly, such feedback can sometimes be terribly generic in content and not very helpful, but occasionally you do get a clear statement of what your application lacked.

Although medical places shouldn't appear in UCAS Clearing, as Medicine typically doesn't participate in Clearing, check as a formality anyway. Clearing is the final matching service offered through UCAS, available after A-level results are published. More realistically, if you have no offers or didn't get the grades your conditional offer demands, and you still desperately want to be a doctor without studying another subject as an undergraduate, you have no option but to reapply the following year.

Reapplying to medical school

At this stage, you need to be realistic. Look at your grades, test scores, exam predictions and extracurricular activities: most likely one (or several) of them wasn't quite strong enough first time round. Feedback from your medical schools can help narrow down which areas let you down. If you intend to reapply, identify the weak link and strengthen it.

If you receive a conditional offer to medical school but don't get the grades, phone the admissions department of your medical school immediately. Some schools have a small amount of leeway if you only just miss out and others may hold your place for you while you re-sit A-levels. Don't just assume that you've lost your place!

If you don't get any offers or your medical school isn't willing to bend on the grade requirement, you have to reapply.

If you get no offers, you do have one advantage: by the time you reapply, you'll have your A-level results. In the time between the end of the application process and sitting your A-levels, study as if you have more to prove than everyone else and let yourself feel just a little bit angry about that situation, because doing so motivates you to prove the world wrong.

The big risk is that your disappointment results in simply giving up on your A-levels, which definitely prevents you from becoming a doctor.

When you get your A-level results, begin the process of researching medical schools again. You may have to change your application choices as a reapplying student, because not all medical schools accept reapplications and the official information they provide doesn't always reflect the nuances for those that do. Your optimal strategy is to contact the schools you're interested in and ask their advice.

Beef up your work experience, re-sit any tests required (for example UKCAT, which we cover in Chapters 6 and 7) and think about how to make the most of your accidental gap year. You need to do something productive with a majority of the available time. Not all your chosen activities have to be medically-related, but consider foreign travel, charity work and getting a part-time job, especially in a medically-related field. Don't just sit on your backside playing video games!

The underlying point is that everything you do in this period needs to be 'sell-able' on your next UCAS personal statement, making you a better candidate for medical school than before.

 Reapplying isn't a dead end. Many students successfully get into medical school the second time around. The successful ones channel their disappointment and anger into productive activity. As a result they get better grades and higher test scores, do more work experience and generally use the setback to motivate them to strive harder.

Of course, you have to decide if medicine really means that much to you. If you truly want to be a doctor and in your heart of hearts know that you have what it takes, you can think of missing out on a place the first time as poor luck and as an opportunity to refine your application. On the other hand, if deep down you don't really care that much about medicine and applied originally out of social pressure (or you know that your grades are never going to be good enough), the setback can be an opportunity for you to consider what you want to do with life, and that's also a very important task.

 Don't rush into a decision; these are big life questions and so take time to think carefully. And when you decide, commit thoroughly to your strategy. That way, whatever happens, you'll have few regrets.

Thinking about studying abroad

If you can't get into a UK medical school and money isn't an issue, you may want to consider studying abroad at a private medical school. If you're in this situation, check out Chapter 2, where we cover the pros and cons of studying overseas.

Part IV
The Part of Tens

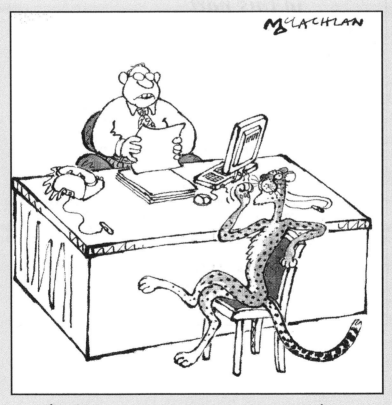

'Right — you were pretty good on the
speed tests — now we come to the
intelligence test ....'

In this part...

Every *For Dummies* book ends with a Part of Tens. It's a chance for us to give you some tips that we couldn't quite fit into the rest of the text.

Medical school applications are highly competitive, and so standing out from the crowd is key. You don't need to be the best candidate in the world to get into a UK medical school; you just need to be better than most of your competition. Chapter 15 contains our top ten tips on standing out from the crowd.

We realise that all this competition is stressful. In Chapter 16, we list ten effective techniques for managing the stress or anxiety that you may be feeling as a result of applying to medical school. These techniques are life skills that will serve you well throughout your career in medicine.

We believe that you can get into medical school and that the tips in this part will give you an edge over your competition.

Chapter 15

Ten Great Ways to Stand Out from the Crowd

. . . .

In This Chapter

▶ Preparing and revising thoroughly

▶ Catching the eye of medical schools

. . . .

*L*ots of great students apply to study medicine and so getting into medical school is all about standing out from the crowd. Successful applicants somehow manage to distinguish themselves from the rest of the field.

To help you do likewise, we provide ten ways to give your application the best possible chance of success.

Starting to Prepare Early

The sooner you do the research on medicine as a career and make a firm decision about whether it's right for you, the better.

An early start gives you more time to plan your work experience, revise for exams and selection tests, and begin to think about your personal statement (which we describe in Chapter 5). As a result you're likely to perform better at all these tasks, and stand out from those who decide to apply to medical school only at the last minute.

 Obviously, we don't suggest setting your heart on a career in medicine from too early an age; that can be unrealistic. But by the time you're finishing up your GCSEs or just starting on your A-levels, you should have a fair idea about whether you want to study medicine at university.

Analysing Your Strengths and Weaknesses

Not everyone is cut out to be a doctor. Think carefully about your character and personality and ask whether you'll enjoy the life of a doctor. Medicine can be a lot of fun but it's also a very demanding job and if you don't think that you're going to relish the experience, you're wiser to pick something else. Chapter 1 of this book has lots of information about the pros and cons of medicine as a career.

Also, think honestly about your academic ability: are you going to get good enough grades and can you perform well on selection tests such as the UKCAT and BMAT (check out Chapters 6 and 8, respectively)? A little bit of soul-searching at the start can save you a great deal of heartache in the longer term, and importantly help identify your strengths and weaknesses.

Possessing good insight is the first step to being able to make good decisions, a skill that doctors need. It also allows you to talk intelligently and rationally about your decision to study medicine, which means that you create a stronger personal statement (turn to Chapter 5) and perform better at interviews (which we discuss in Part III), as well as giving you extra motivation to study hard.

Getting Your Personal Statement Right

Your personal statement in your application is crucial; it's the only thing that university shortlisters really have to distinguish you from the rest of your competition. So start drafting your statement early, and read and revise it multiple times. Then put it away in a drawer and come back to it a month or two later. Revise it again in light of the work experience you've done in the meantime.

In others words, work on your personal statement in the same way you'd work for an exam.

Chapter 5 contains lots of advice on how to write a good personal statement. Read it carefully.

Accepting That Work Experience Matters

Almost everyone applying to medical school is going to get top-notch grades, but not everyone has top-notch work experience. This is one of the best ways to stand out from the crowd.

Think about what medical schools want to see from potential doctors and choose work experience that demonstrates these talents. Try to get a variety of placements, from the more glamorous side of medicine to the nitty-gritty of the coal-face. We provide loads more info in Chapter 4.

Most importantly, think actively about what you learn from your work experience and try to put that down in words. Concentrate on what it told you about yourself and about medicine, and how the two are related. Include these points in the drafts of your personal statement and think about how to summarise them concisely for your interview.

In addition, think about one or two scenarios from your work experience to use if interviewers go down the behavioural interviewing route and ask about how you reacted to past challenging situations, or may react to future hypothetical ones. We cover behavioural interviewing in Chapter 12.

Revising for the Selection Tests

Don't listen to anyone who tells you that you can't revise for tests such as the UKCAT and BMAT. The more familiar you are with these exams, the better you're likely to perform on them. For this reason we run specific courses at www.getintomedicalschool.org and devote space to the tests in Part II's chapters.

A good test score rarely gets you into medical school, but a bad one can certainly keep you out. An exceptionally high score, especially in the BMAT, definitely impresses the universities that require it.

Keeping Up to Date with Medical Matters

Not everyone who applies to medical school knows much about medicine, which quickly becomes obvious when they get asked questions about current medical issues or ethical dilemmas (turn to Chapter 13 for more info). No one expects you to be as familiar with these issues as a good doctor should be, but knowing more about them than your competition impresses interviewers and scores you lots of brownie points.

Good ways of keeping up to date are to read the health sections of the broadsheet newspapers or their websites. We also update a free blog at http://GetIntoMedicineUK.com with some of the biggest health stories of the day, as well as make suggestions for areas to think about that interviewers may discuss.

Practising Interviews

Interviewing well is a skill that improves with practice and yet most medical school applicants have had little opportunity to become good interviewees.

A good interview performance separates you from the herd. Chapter 11 has a lot of information on how to perform well in an interview setting. You can try practising with friends, or with a teacher/careers adviser who knows what they're talking about at your school. A kindly GP may be willing to give you some interview practice too. Alternatively, courses are available to hone your interview skills through practice sessions, mock interviews and structured feedback to improve your technique.

Other ways to practise include verbally summarising topics and trying to persuade other people of your point of view, for example in a school debating club. Thinking more laterally, you can get an opportunity to practise these skills in a live way if you work in a part-time or weekend sales job.

Staying Cool under Pressure

Keeping calm lets you focus on dealing with whatever challenge you're facing without being distracted by tension. Using stress positively is also something you need to do as a great doctor.

Being cool under pressure results in better test scores, stronger interview performances and appearing better than your competition. Chapter 16 has more advice on coping with stress, but also remember that all the other candidates are in the same boat as you; you need only to outperform them marginally to get your place in medical school.

Discerning What Makes You Unique

You probably already have something that makes you stand out from the crowd. The challenge is identifying it and spinning that talent in a direction that demonstrates suitability to a career in medicine.

Try thinking laterally about all the activities you do and enjoy, and ask yourself whether any of them hone skills that doctors require. If some cover similar ground, you're well on your way to creating a distinctive message. Chapter 5 has lots of advice on how to sell yourself appropriately in your personal statement.

Of course, if you just happen to have a genuinely remarkable personal history, by all means finesse that into evidence of potential to be a doctor. For example, if you've represented your country in a junior sporting category, think about all the leadership, team-working and communication skills you've gained.

Avoiding Standing Out in the Wrong Way

You want to stand out by being exceptionally talented, well-rounded and professional. You don't want to be the girl with a dodgy, quasi-criminal past or the guy in the bright orange suit. Doctors have to be ethically sound, responsible-looking, professional people.

Personal expression is a wonderful thing, but during the medical school application process you have to target your presentation to meet the expectations of medical schools. So think about what kind of person they want and present yourself in that light.

Every snowflake may well be unique, but only certain snowflakes are incorporated into the medical school snowball!

Chapter 16

Ten Top Tips for Coping with Stress

In This Chapter
▶ Applying to medical school is stressful
▶ Coping with stress increases your chance of success

*N*o point denying it: the medical school application process is long, complicated and potentially very stressful. In our opinion it's probably unduly burdensome with too many separate hurdles, but the reality is that the process is unlikely to become more streamlined any time soon. Your challenge is to stay calm and cope with the stress so that you perform as well as possible.

We outline ten ways to continue enjoying life while getting into medical school.

Keeping the Big Picture in Mind

Remember that becoming a doctor isn't the sum total of your life experience. Of course, that desire is important to you right now but that doesn't mean it's always going to be so all-consuming. Billions of people manage to live happy, productive and fulfilling lives without being doctors!

Fretting about what happens if you don't get into medical school is natural and can be a major challenge to your self-esteem. But you'd still have lots of other options and potential.

By keeping a sense of perspective about the process, you can take a little bit of the weight off your shoulders and focus calmly on doing well on each step of your application.

Staying Motivated

Stress arises when people feel as if they have no control over what they're doing. Humans evolved flight-or-fight reactions to cope with situations like being attacked by a sabre-toothed tiger. In the modern world, the adrenaline rush turns inwards and makes your mind race and body tense, resulting in stress.

 You have a choice about applying to medical school. You're voluntarily putting yourself under this stress, because the potential outcome is something you want to achieve: being a doctor. You retain ultimate control over the process in the sense that you're choosing this path for yourself. Acknowledging this fundamental truth places the centre of control back in your hands and away from the application system. Your future is yours to decide.

Stress levels naturally reduce when you regain a sense of control and choice about your life decisions.

Taking the Long View

Think about when you're going to be working and when you'll be relaxing, and try to stick to these separated times.

Drawing up a timetable can help you feel in control. Use the medical school application timeline in Chapter 3 as the basis of a more personalised plan of attack. Don't be neurotic about it, though. Your plan needs to cover your time in enough detail to give you a sense of direction, but not so much that it feels suffocating.

Breathing Deeply to Stay Calm

When you're feeling stressed, your body reacts accordingly: the so-called flight-or-fight reaction. Your pulse quickens, your muscles tense up and your breathing becomes faster and shallower. The good news is that this is a two-way relationship; if you notice these changes and act to control them, you can make yourself feel calmer. By consciously slowing down your breathing, and making each breath deeper and more controlled, you can calm and focus your thoughts.

 Try breathing in deeply through your nose and out slowly through slightly pursed lips, taking about five seconds to complete an entire cycle. You don't need to time it; just breathe a little more slowly than normal but not so slow that you're uncomfortable.

The first time you try this technique, you may well lose concentration after a few breaths, but if you keep practising you get better. Eventually, doing it when stressed becomes second nature. The technique can work wonders in relaxing both mind and body.

Relaxing Your Muscles Progressively

When stressed, you can try consciously relaxing your muscles to reduce the tension that prolonged stress builds up in them. You do so by alternately tensing and relaxing your muscles under conscious control. For instance, start off by scrunching up your feet, holding them tensed for a few seconds, and then letting them gradually relax over another few seconds. Repeat the cycle a few times. Then move onto your calf muscles, your thighs, your fists, arms and so on. The whole sequence can take some minutes but that's a good thing, because the task gives you a break from worrying.

Like the deep, controlled breathing from the preceding section, this technique improves with practice, so keep at it.

Visualising for Success

You can use visualisation techniques for relaxation and for confidence-building:

- ✔ **Relaxation:** Close your eyes, think of a time and place where you were at your happiest and try to recall all the physical, sensory and emotional details of the event. Relive it as closely and fully as you can.

- ✔ **Confidence-building:** Focus on a successful outcome. Put yourself in the position of passing your exams with flying colours and getting into medical school, or qualifying from there as a doctor.

Some people feel that this latter exercise is 'tempting fate'. But that opinion is frequently a manifestation of a fear of failure and is best challenged instead of being left to fester unseen in your subconscious. Aim for success, and give yourself inner permission to be a successful person.

Working Hard to Combat Anxiety

The unknown is terrifying and you can project your deepest and darkest fears into that empty space. If you haven't revised and practised properly, fear of the unknown can overwhelm you. But familiarising yourself with all the elements of the application process makes you feel comfortable with the steps you need to take. That very familiarity then acts as a reassuring, soothing protective shield around you.

The information in this book helps you realise that the application process is large but manageable. It's not easy, but thousands of people complete it successfully. Absolutely no reason exists why you can't be one of them.

Work hard to revise for your exams and other tests, and do plenty of practice for your interviews. You won't regret the effort.

Refusing to Run Away

Stress and anxiety are normal parts of life and medical school applications, but that doesn't mean you can't control them. The tips in this chapter can help you do that.

Don't try to run away from the pressure. For instance, don't be tempted to use alcohol or drugs to block it out. Such attempts never work in the long term, and just lead to more problems and distress.

Confronting and dealing with your stresses is always preferable to ignoring or avoiding them.

Sparing Your Friends and Family

When you're feeling stressed, taking out that pent-up frustration on others is all too easy, and it usually ends up being on those closest to you. Try not to let this happen too often; use the techniques in this chapter instead.

Your friends and family love you and will forgive you to some extent, but you'll still feel guilty about it. Better to use other ways of de-stressing.

Giving Yourself a Break

Remember that the medical school application process is a marathon, not a sprint. If you work at 100 per cent effort throughout it, you simply burn yourself out. Ensure that you take time out to do the things you love doing and be with the people you like. As a result you unwind and relax, and are much more effective when the time comes to work again.

Good luck, and try to have fun too. You can do it!

Index

About the Authors

Dr Chris Chopdar is co-founder of Get into Medical School Ltd, which has a strong track record of getting prospective medical students into the university of their choice. He enjoys teaching its courses both in Oxford and at schools and colleges across the UK. Chris got his medical degree from Oxford University and also has a Master's degree in Physiological Sciences from his time there.

He returned to Oxford as a psychiatrist after brief stints working in other parts of the country. Chris continues in clinical practice, combining this work with interests in interview technique and the psychological motifs inherent in clothing.

Dr Neel Burton is co-founder of Get into Medical School Ltd, designed its UKCAT course and also coaches individual UKCAT candidates. Having qualified in Medicine from the University of London, he is now a psychiatrist, philosopher and writer.

Neel lives and teaches in Oxford, where he also runs the Oxford Wine Academy and the Meaning of Madness course. He is recipient of the Society of Authors' Richard Asher Prize, the British Medical Association's Young Authors' Award and the Medical Journalists' Association Open Book Award. He's happy to talk at charities, schools, universities and other public gatherings.

More information on **Get into Medical School**, and the courses it offers, can be found at www.getintomedicalschool.org.

Authors' Acknowledgements

Author Henry David Thoreau said, *'It's not what you look at that matters, but what you see.'*

We're grateful that Mike Baker, our commissioning editor, could see the potential of a *For Dummies* book helping students get into medical school. Erica Peters, our project editor, brought this vision to life and the entire Wiley team — especially Andy Finch — were similarly eagle-eyed throughout the production process. Special thanks go to Dr Tom Stockmann and Dr Pat Lindley, whose insightful suggestions have undoubtedly enhanced the book.

This book is the product of many months of concerted effort; getting into medical school also requires much effort. Dummies don't get into medical school but we believe that the simple, clear and logical *For Dummies* approach will make your preparation easier.

Good luck!

Dedication

We dedicate this book to prospective medical students everywhere.
We wish you flourishing careers and happy lives.

Publisher's Acknowledgements

We're proud of this book; please send us your comments at http://dummies.custhelp.com. For other comments, please contact our Customer Care Department within the U.S. at 877-762-2974, outside the U.S. at (001) 317-572-3993, or fax 317-572-4002.

Some of the people who helped bring this book to market include the following:

Acquisitions, Editorial, and Vertical Websites

Project Editor: Erica Peters

Commissioning Editor: Mike Baker

Assistant Editor: Ben Kemble

Development Editor: Andy Finch

Technical Reviewers: Dr Tom Stockmann, Dr Pat Lindley

Copy Editor: Kate O'Leary

Proofreader: Martin Key

Production Manager: Daniel Mersey

Publisher: Miles Kendall

Cover Photo: © dra_schwartz / iStock

Cartoons: Ed McLachlan

Composition Services

Senior Project Coordinator: Kristie Rees

Layout and Graphics: Carrie Cesavice, Jennifer Creasey, Amy Hassos, Jennifer Henry, Christin Swinford

Proofreader: Dwight Ramsey

Indexer: Potomac Indexing, LLC

Special Help

Brand Reviewer: Jennifer Bingham

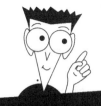

FOR DUMMIES

Making Everything Easier! ™

FOR STUDENTS

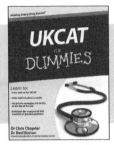

978-1-119-96584-8

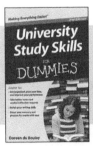

978-1-118-31548-4

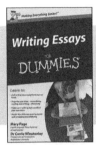

978-0-470-74290-7

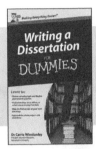

978-0-470-74270-9

SCIENCE & MATHS

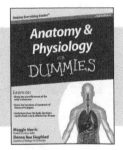

978-0-470-92326-9

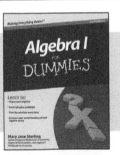

978-0-470-55964-2

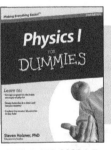

978-0-470-90324-7

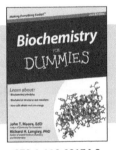

978-1-118-02174-3

HOBBIES

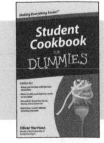

978-0-470-74711-7

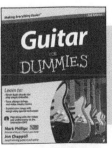

978-1-118-11554-1

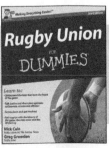

978-1-119-99092-5

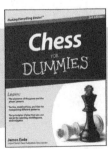

978-1-118-01695-4

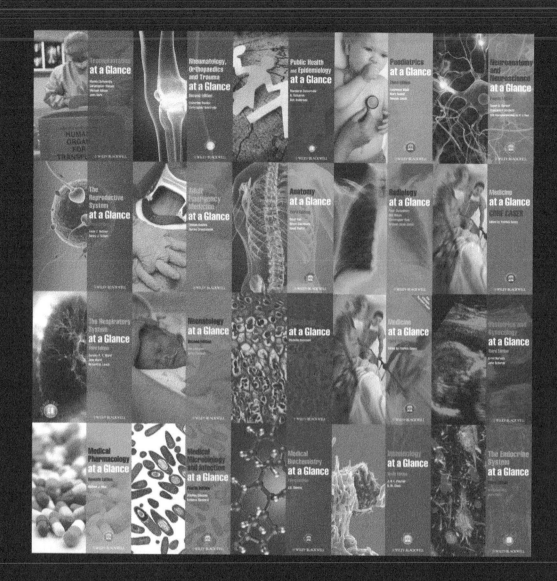

The at a Glance series

Popular double-page spread format • Coverage of core knowledge
Full-colour throughout • Self-assessment to test your knowledge • Expert authors

www.wileymedicaleducation.com

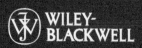